Pregnant Women on Drugs

Pregnant Women on Drugs

Combating Stereotypes and Stigma

Sheigla Murphy
Marsha Rosenbaum

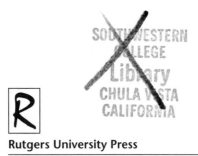

Rutgers University Press

New Brunswick, New Jersey, and London

Library of Congress Cataloging-in-Publication Data

Murphy, Sheigla, 1949–
     Pregnant women on drugs : combating stereotypes and stigma /
Sheigla Murphy and Marsha Rosenbaum.
          p.   cm.
     Includes bibliographical references and index.
     ISBN 0–8135–2602–7 (hardcover : alk. paper). —
ISBN 0–8135–2603–5 (pbk. : alk. paper)
     1. Pregnant women—Drug use—Interviews.   2. Drug abuse in
pregnancy.   I. Rosenbaum, Marsha, 1948–   .   II. Title.
HV5824.W6M87   1999
362.29'12'082—dc21   98–20130
                                                                        CIP

British Cataloging-in-Publication data for this book is available from
the British Library

Manufactured in the United States of America

To my daughters, Moira and Sarah O'Neil

Sheigla Murphy

To my children: Jeanette, Katy, Anne, and Johnny Irwin

Marsha Rosenbaum

Contents

Acknowledgments

This book is the result of the contributions of many people who deserve not only recognition but our deepest gratitude. We are most indebted to the study participants who shared with us their personal and often painful stories. This book would not have been possible without the cooperation of these courageous women, who gave their time and bared their souls in an effort to help others.

Margaret Kearney and Katherine Irwin conducted interviews and participated in our weekly analysis sessions, where the beginnings of a conceptual framework emerged. Dr. Kearney selected the crack users' interviews for her dissertation research and published articles on prenatal care, sex, and fertility and a grounded theory of the self during crack-involved pregnancies in *Contemporary Drug Problems, Social Science and Medicine, Nursing Research*, and *Qualitative Health Research*. Katherine Irwin's work, drawing on the narratives of the entire study sample (published in *Contemporary Drug Problems*), explores the intersection of the ideological context and individual experience. Kimberly Theidon joined the project staff toward the end of the second year. She participated in later analysis sessions as well as the preparation of the final report for the National Institute on Drug Abuse along with Jeanette Irwin. Ms. Theidon's article reporting the findings from her analysis of the role of violence in pregnant drug users' lives was also published in *Contemporary Drug Problems*. All of these articles are referenced throughout the book, and complete citations are located in the reference list.

We appreciate the efforts of Rhoda Nussbaum, M.D., who acted as our medical consultant, and Lynn Wenger, who located potential participants and conducted the social workers' interviews. John Irwin assisted with the analysis of the demographic data. Brandy Britton and Rebecca Wepsic conducted several interviews and attended early analysis sessions. We thank our brother and colleague, Craig Reinarman, for countless long and constructive phone calls from the beginning of the proposal writing process until our final submission to Rutgers.

The funding provided by the National Institute on Drug Abuse made this project possible. We appreciate the encouragement of Dr. Jag Khalsa, and we owe a special debt to Dr. Coryl Jones for her considerable enthusiasm, advice, and support. Thanks also to the staff at Scientific Analysis Corporation, Setsu Gee, Dr. Dorothy Miller, and Sandie Spacek, who provided us with the requisite resources and a supportive working environment.

Administrative assistants Sharon Michalske and Sue Eldredge gave tirelessly of their time. Ms. Michalske helped with data management and initial analyses as well as completing screening interviews with potential interviewees. During 1997–98, the commitment and professionalism of both Ms. Michalske and Ms. Eldredge were invaluable throughout the many rewrites and revisions required to turn numerous drafts into a publication.

We thank Moira O'Neil for her excellent editorial as well as substantive comments on earlier versions and Lynn Zimmer, our friend and colleague, who devoted many hours to writing carefully crafted comments and criticisms of the (not quite) final draft. Martha Heller (and the staff at Rutgers University Press) was an ongoing source of inspiration, motivation, and editorial help. We believe the book was much improved by each of these women's generous and thoughtful contributions.

Finally, our families and friends deserve special thanks for their unflagging love and support. We are particularly grateful for their patience and continued belief in the importance of our work. All of the people we have acknowledged deserve credit for everything that is good in this book.

Pregnant Women on Drugs

1

Wayward

Wombs

When people believe the hand that rocks the cradle would rather be smoking rocks, diverse constituencies unite in moral outrage and condemnation. For most people, the image of a mother purposefully hurting her helpless fetus conjures extremely negative feelings and reactions. In modern society the use of illegal drugs during pregnancy is commonly defined as the antithesis of responsible behavior and good health. The two statuses, pregnant woman and drug user, simply do not go together.

A pregnant woman is supposed to take care of and protect her forming fetus. Women who purposely poison their wombs by using drugs are seen as failing in their reproductive role, and they must take their place among the most stigmatized groups in modern society. Yet thousands of women of childbearing age use illegal drugs, and a smaller group continues to do so while pregnant. Krista's story illustrates the types of life experiences that often lead to drug-involved pregnancies.[1]

When we met Krista, she was six months' pregnant. Krista was introduced to pot laced with PCP when she was nine years old and began using speed when she was twelve.

Her drug use escalated after she was raped at fifteen and began using heroin. Krista gave birth to five children and lost custody of all of them because the police caught her children panhandling. She had difficulty expressing her sadness because "It's not a matter of words, it's a matter of feelings." When the police questioned Krista about her drug use, she answered them honestly: "By doing that, my whole life changed. By being honest and telling them, 'Yes, I do drugs,' and trying to work something out with the system, to get on a program, to get my kids back and the whole game they play, things got worse and worse."

Her children were placed in foster care far from the city where she lived, and Krista was never able to make the three-hour bus trip to visit them. Because she had not visited them in more than a year, the children's social worker declared Krista an uncaring and uninterested mother. The children were put up for adoption.

Krista was hopeful about becoming a mother again. She described her current partner as "wonderful":

> I'm amazed after all this bad luck I've had to actually find a person in this world that is for me. I didn't think it was possible. I thought everybody was really screwed up. But I'm going to give life one more chance. I'm gonna try. I've already got a name for the baby, no matter if this is a boy or a girl. The baby's middle name is Ember. And what that means is the last fire of hope for me. Ember, like the ember of a fire.

As a result of her failings with her older children, Krista saw her current pregnancy as an opportunity to "give life one more chance," a chance to start over and to be a better mother this time. When we interviewed Krista, and 119 other women, we wanted to understand the experiences and perspectives of pregnant drug users. Most of the women we

talked with had one or two older children and were expect-
ing or had recently given birth to a newborn. Yet Krista's
view of her pregnancy exemplifies that of many other
interviewees. Impending birth represented choosing life, an
opportunity for redemption for past failures, hopes for the
future, and a chance to claim a socially acceptable and respectable identity.

As Krista said so eloquently, Ember was her "last fire of
hope."

We titled this chapter "Wayward Wombs" for two reasons: first, *wombs* represent our feminist perspective that
women continue to be defined by their reproductive functions; second, *wayward* connotes the deviant drug-using
behaviors that moved our interviewees away from socially
acceptable identities and roles. It is important to review the
literature on pregnancy, drug use, and drug treatment to
locate our findings in a historical context. We must also
examine the impact of the 1980s–90s war on drugs—more
specifically, on pregnant drug users.

Women on Heroin

Drug use during pregnancy has concerned physicians
and scientists since they began to treat and study this problematic phenomenon. The 1960s and 1970s marked a decided increase in the available scientific literature on the
effects of opiate use during pregnancy. Heroin addiction was
thought to be connected with problems such as premature
rupture of membranes, impaired fetal growth, diminished
birth weight, preterm delivery, maternal infections, meconium staining, stillbirths, toxemia, and infant withdrawal
(Blinick 1971; Blinick, Wallach, and Jerez 1969; Finnegan
1975, 1979; Glass 1974; Kandall et al. 1976; Naeye et al.
1973; Naeye, Ladis, and Drage 1976; Ostrea, Chavez, and

Strauss 1976; Rementeria and Nunag 1973; Stone, Salerna, and Green 1971; Wilson et al. 1979; Zelson 1973; Zelson, Rubio, and Wasserman 1989; Zuspan et al. 1975).

Our own interest in pregnancy and drug use coincided with the proliferation of information in the mid-1970s. We first studied heroin addiction in 1977 as part of a study funded by the National Institute on Drug Abuse (NIDA) entitled "The Career of the Woman Addict." During the course of this research, we interviewed one hundred women, 70 percent of whom were mothers. Since our study was sociological and ethnographic as well as focused on the women rather than fetal outcomes, our findings differed from the more medical- and fetal outcomes–oriented works just referenced.

Discovery of pregnancy was problematic because many women stopped menstruating when they were addicted. By the time they acknowledged their pregnancies (often because they were showing), they were often more than sixteen weeks pregnant. Many women felt they were too far along to obtain an abortion. It was also too late to stop using drugs because heroin's most deleterious effects occur during the first trimester, and withdrawal in later stages of pregnancy is too dangerous for the fetus.

Birth and delivery, according to our study participants, were often physiologically as well as psychologically difficult. Many of the women suffered from ailments such as toxemia and spotty (if any) prenatal care attendance. Consequently, for most heroin-using women, birth was a dangerous and fearful experience. Additionally, when hospital staff were aware of the women's drug use, they became less than supportive and often abusive. The last thing the women wanted to do was to return to such an unpleasant environment, and some never came back. To compound the hospital staff's disdainful expressions, women frequently went home with an irritable and difficult infant. This combination often launched their mothering careers with feelings of failure and provided an impetus to use heroin to relieve their guilt and alleviate suffering (Rosenbaum 1981).

Treatment for the Pregnant Addict

During the 1970s, the term *pregnant addict* was equated with pregnant heroin users. Scientists and interventionists began to perceive pregnant drug users as a special population of addicts, largely due to their childbearing and child-rearing roles. Treatment options for heroin-addicted women were limited, with methadone maintenance treatment (MMT) the major modality available. At that time, research on MMT and pregnancy focused on medical issues pertaining to the fetus and the newborn and the management of the pregnant addict (Blinick, Jerez, and Wallach 1973; Blinick et al. 1975; Clark et al. 1974; Cohen and Neumann 1973; Connaughton et al. 1974, 1977; Davis and Chappel 1973; Finnegan 1978; Finnegan, Connaughton, and Emich 1972; Harper et al. 1974; Kandall et al. 1976; Newman 1974; Rajegowda et al. 1972; Ramer and Lodge 1975; Statzer and Wardell 1966; Sullivan, Fischbach, and Hornick 1972; Waldeman 1973; Wallach, Jerez, and Blinick 1969; Zelson, Lee, and Casalino 1973; Zelson and Sook 1973; Zuspan et al. 1975). Research findings, while generally supportive of methadone as a harm-reduction tool, were inconsistent in terms of infant health and severity of withdrawal symptoms. Still, for a pregnant addict who found it impossible to quit using heroin, maintenance was one of the few viable options; and by the end of the 1970s, women occupied nearly one-third of the new MMT slots (Arif and Westermeyer 1990).

Our interest in drug treatment for women began with

our study of women heroin addicts. We found MMT to be an increasingly integral component of heroin users' worlds. Heroin-using women had to confront the possibility of getting on methadone, whether or not they chose to enroll in a program. For this reason, we embarked on another NIDA-funded study, "The Methadone Experience for Women." During the course of that project, we learned a great deal about what drug treatment was like for pregnant women and mothers.

We found the discovery of pregnancy encouraged some women to enroll in methadone programs (Rosenbaum 1982). The women who enrolled in MMT opted for the external controls the program provided. Their lives were necessarily stabilized due to the highly structured clinic routine and their decreased need to participate in criminal activities to pay for heroin. Methadone patients' lives became much more routinized, enabling the women to focus on things other than attending to their addiction, such as providing a home for their baby, eating well, and learning the requisite parenting skills.

Despite enlisting in drug treatment and attempting to stabilize their lives, many women reported that when they went to the hospital to give birth, they were faced with the stigma of being "just a junkie." The guilt that they may have been able to suppress during pregnancy often resurfaced when dealing with the hostility of health care workers.

The guilt experienced by women on methadone surfaced in the hospital but did not end there. Women reported feeling responsible for the baby's withdrawal, although there was no way to predict severity of withdrawal or even whether or not it would occur (Finnegan, Connaughton, and Emich 1973; Lodge, Marcus, and Ramer 1975; Mondanaro 1977; Rajegowda et al. 1972; Reddy, Harper, and Stern 1971; Zelson 1973).

Motherhood often began badly for methadone-addicted women, and there were even more problems when they brought the baby home from the hospital. Just as with heroin, babies in methadone withdrawal could be extremely irritable (Lodge 1975; Mondanaro 1977). Interviewees with withdrawing infants described their postpartum depression as exacerbated and extended. Seemingly never-ending guilt haunted mothers on methadone. First, they looked for signs that their babies were addicted. Later, women wondered if their children's problems were caused by their heroin and/ or methadone use. The women with grown children reported that this guilt and fear extended throughout their children's lives, with every ailment suspect.

Women and Cocaine

By the mid-1980s, cocaine had replaced heroin as the "most dangerous" drug. A number of cross-sectional surveys documented the dramatic rise in incidence and prevalence of cocaine use and its related problems (Abelson and Miller 1985; Adams and Durell 1984; Fishburne, Abelson, and Cisin 1979; Greene, Nightingale, and DuPont 1975; Inciardi 1986; Johnston, Bachman, and O'Malley 1984). Generally, women's drug use seemed to be increasing (NIDA 1987), particularly among women of childbearing age (Clayton et al. 1985). There was a paucity of research on cocaine-using women themselves. As with heroin, the bulk of the scientific literature focused on sexuality, sexual function (Siegel 1982), pregnancy, fetal development, and neonatal behavior (Acker et al. 1983; Newald 1986). At that time, most research on women's cocaine use was derived from case studies with very small samples or from large surveys in which women were peripheral (Carr 1975; Deren 1986; Kaestner et al. 1986). The increase in the number of young women smoking the then new drug, crack, became a serious concern. Numerous media articles indicated a growing awareness of crack cocaine–smoking women among health and treatment professionals. Of particular concern was the expanding involvement of young mothers or pregnant women in crack-using scenes. Greater numbers of women were seeking treatment for crack cocaine dependence with a corresponding rise in reports of cocaine-involved pregnancies, child abuse, and abandonment.

Although incidence, prevalence, and epidemiological data on women and cocaine existed in the mid to late 1980s, etiological and ethnographic research was sorely lacking. In 1989, we embarked on our own sociological NIDA–funded study of one hundred women who used crack cocaine, sixty-eight of whom were mothers at the time of interview.

We found that women crack users' early lives set the stage for later crack use:

> Early in life, many were trapped by childhoods in violent, fragmented, or drug-involved households; teenage pregnancies; truncated educations and lack of skills; poverty that was worsened by diversion of resources to drugs; oppressive relationships with men; and, eventually, by the demeaning social world surrounding crack cocaine. (Kearney, Murphy, and Rosenbaum 1994a, 147)

The women's viewpoints on pregnancy had much to do with their general world views, structured by life experiences. Interviewees believed they were controlled by chance rather than their own life choices. Many believed babies, rather than a chosen responsibility, were gifts "from God." Controlling birth was a distant issue rather than a present reality and distinct possibility. Unprotected sexual experiences were attributed to youth, lack of knowledge, power-lessness, carelessness, or ambivalence. The trauma of rape often increased their vulnerability and fatalism. As a conse-quence of women's beliefs and unforeseen experiences, most became pregnant unexpectedly (Kearney, Murphy, and Rosenbaum 1994a). Women told us they had wanted to be mothers at some point in their lives, even if they did not determine when exactly this should occur. Lacking the op-portunities to assume other viable social roles involving educational or occupational pursuits, they found that moth-erhood remained one of the few conventional, respectable life options.

The crack-using women in our study did not resemble the uncaring, unfeeling monsters portrayed in the popular media at that time (Kearney, Murphy, and Rosenbaum 1994b; Irwin 1995; Murphy forthcoming; Rosenbaum et al. 1990). On the contrary, they felt a strong responsibility for their children as well as deep shame when they failed. Like other mothers, they expressed maternal goals of nurturing and positive modeling. Crack cocaine use presented serious problems, including a lack of attention to children's physi-cal and emotional needs, a drain on household finances, and negative role modeling. Women found themselves in a down-ward spiral as crack intoxication momentarily alleviated guilty maternal feelings, which ultimately worsened the situation. Nonetheless, some women carved out various strategies in an effort to maintain some semblance of moth-ering standards while continuing to use crack. They tried to separate drug use from parental responsibilities, budgeted money, and tried to get away from the crack scene. Many reluctantly but voluntarily relinquished their children for their own good to a more responsible party. When custody was lost, whether voluntarily or involuntarily, most women used even more crack; for as one woman eloquently expressed her feelings of loss and self-blame, "When they took my babies, they took myself" (Kearney, Murphy, and Rosenbaum 1994b, 256; Murphy forthcoming).

By the early 1990s, we had completed three research projects on women's drug use. Whether we were studying heroin, methadone, or cocaine, it was apparent that pregnancy and motherhood were controversial and difficult issues. The drug treatment field was beginning to acknowledge women and children's unique problems. This acknowledgment, however, was not accompanied by the allocation of enough real resources or the creation of effective interventions. By the mid-1980s, President and Mrs. Reagan's War on Drugs was underway, which negatively affected an already seriously problematic situation.

In the midst of what was characterized by policymakers and politicians as a war on drug use, the image of the crack baby was born. Incited by rhetoric about the so-called crack cocaine epidemic described by numerous other social analysts (Beckett 1995; Humphries et al. 1992; Lieb and Sterk-Elifson 1995; Reinarman and Levine 1989), observers predicted that the crack mother and her compromised progeny would topple the swollen national health care budget and dismantle the American school system.

The Crack Scare

Unwittingly, Ira Chasnoff (1989) estimated that there were 375,000 crack-involved pregnancies and set off a media-fueled panic about the out-of-control epidemic of cocaine use during pregnancy. The popular press wrote hundreds of stories about the problems of babies exposed to crack in utero. For example, in one newspaper story, crack babies were predicted to "present an overwhelming challenge to schools, future employers and society" (Blakeslee 1989, 1).

Crack use was said to "overwhelm one of the strongest forces in nature, the parental instinct" (Hinds 1990, 9); drug use during pregnancy was "interfering with the central core of what it is to be human" (Blakeslee 1989, 1). Negative media attention on drugs reached an all-time peak with the creation of the crack baby phenomenon (Irwin 1995; Glasser and Siegel 1997; Morgan and Zimmer 1997; Reinarman and Levine 1989; Siegel 1997). When preliminary research findings indicated that crack use during pregnancy might be associated with fetal morbidity, the popular press quickly ran a series of alarmist stories. Journalists reported that crack cocaine–addicted mothers had utter disregard for their children (*New York Times*, 1990). Crack made a mother "indifferent to her child or abusive when its cries irritate her" (*Economist*, 1989, 28). The use of drugs—specifically, crack use—during pregnancy became equivalent to abusive parenting since crack use was said to sever "that deepest and most sacred of bonds: that between a mother and child" (Gillman 1989, 3).

Criminal Justice Responses

As a result of media extrapolations of preliminary or unreplicated findings, pregnant drug users suffered greater stigmatization and were further marginalized. As if the situation was not already bad enough for drug-using women and their children, in the early 1990s the justice system stepped in and attempted to criminalize drug use during pregnancy (Humphries et al. 1992; McNulty 1987; Siegel 1997). Prosecutors in twenty-three states entered the arena, employing a punitive solution: criminal prosecution (Balisy 1987; Norton-Hawk 1994; Paltrow 1992; Siegel 1990; Vega et al. 1993). A drug-using pregnant woman faced arrest and potential incarceration for delivering drugs to a minor. A woman who tested positive for drugs during hospital delivery risked losing custodial rights of her newborn. Although by 1991 the earlier reported relationship between fetal harm and maternal cocaine use had not been replicated by subsequent research (Coles et al. 1992; Koren et al. 1989; Lutiger et al. 1991; Zuckerman 1991), all over the United States, infants and children continued to be removed from their mothers' custody, overwhelming inner-city foster care and child welfare systems.

Voices of Protest

In a move simultaneous to increased public outcry and maternal prosecutions, a small group of academics, attorneys, and researchers began to question the efficacy and fairness of the criminal justice approach to the problem of pregnancy and drug use. They argued that the social conditions of crack users' lives were far more deleterious to a mother and child's health, well-being, and safety than drug use. Further, they claimed that the focus on women's drug use was political, purposeful, and oversimplified. Crack mothers were being scapegoated to divert attention from the realities of the failed, post-Reagan cutbacks of needed social programs to address complex social problems. Some social analysts believed that addressing the real problems underlying pregnancy and drug use would require major changes in existing social and economic arrangements—that is, guaranteed income for mothers and children, national health care, and affordable child care (Reinarman and Levine 1989; Rosenbaum et al. 1990; Siegel 1990; Trebach and Zeese 1990).

Our previous work led us to believe that more information was needed to construct efficacious interventions rather than continue in the harmful direction of persecution, prosecution, and punishment of pregnant drug users. Meanwhile, the prevalence of drug use during pregnancy remained the same (Gomby and Shiono 1991); and low birth weight, small head circumference, irritability, sudden infant deaths, and malformation among babies born to drug-using mothers continued to be reported (Zuckerman et al. 1989).

What was missing from the available knowledge base were studies that focused on women rather than on their offspring. Our goal was to understand the experiences and perspectives of the women who use the hardest drugs, even while they are pregnant.

The Pregnancy and Drug Use Study

The Focus on Women

In 1991, there was a glaring hole in the literature on pregnancy and drug use. While extensive and sophisticated knowledge concerning fetal outcome was available, there was a paucity of information about the mother herself. We did, however, learn from prior research that, compared with nondrug users, the pregnant addict was less likely to attend prenatal care appointments, more likely to live in poor conditions, more likely to have a host of confounding problems such as sexually transmitted diseases, and more likely to experience higher rates of violence (Amaro et al. 1990; Robins and Mills 1993; Weimann, Berenson, and Landwehr 1995; Weimann, Berenson, and San Miguel 1994). Nevertheless, the details of her social world had not been well mapped out. As a result, it remained difficult to understand how each of the factors in a pregnant drug user's life affected and was affected by her drug use as well as the individual and cumulative effects of these factors. This, in turn, limited the ability of medical and drug treatment professionals to provide appropriate obstetrical and drug treatment services.

Given the limitations of the available research, it seemed important to focus on understanding the context of pregnant drug users' lives. In the summer of 1991, we embarked on the "Pregnancy and Drugs" (PAD) study to understand the experience of being a pregnant addict, the decision-making processes regarding discovery and termination/continuation of the pregnancy, drug-use patterns (including routes of administration), the seeking/not seeking of prenatal or drug treatment, and the role of her relationships with significant others (for example, the father, her parents, and her other children). Previously, women's feelings and beliefs about parenting had not been examined outside treatment settings.

Our Choice of Drugs to Study

We interviewed women who used heroin and stimulants—specifically, cocaine, crack, and methamphetamine—during pregnancy. We chose these drugs for several reasons:

1. The use of these substances posed a potential serious health threat to both mother and child.
2. These drugs were frequently injected.
3. Their illicit nature set them apart from other licit and even illicit drugs used during pregnancy (such as alcohol, tobacco, prescription drugs, and marijuana).
4. The drug-related stigma made it less likely that users would seek either prenatal care or drug treatment.

Heroin and stimulants had been previously shown to cause a myriad of deleterious physiological effects on babies who were exposed to them in utero. Compared with other illicit drugs, heroin and stimulants had the greatest impact on infant mortality as well as on other standard measures of infant health (Habel, Kaye, and Lee 1990). Another health hazard disproportionately affecting users of these drugs (and their babies) was exposure to HIV and other needle-borne infections. Heroin and stimulants were more likely to be used intravenously than any of the other illicit drugs, thereby exposing mothers-to-be to the AIDS virus through needle sharing. Finally, heroin and stimulants were expensive and often pushed women into criminal activities and exposed them to their attendant dangers.

Goals of the Study

Our most important goal was to understand the basic social and social-psychological processes that characterized drug use during pregnancy. We believed (and still believe) that, by gathering this information, we would be in a better position to make sound scientific recommendations toward the ultimate goal of instituting humane, pragmatic policies to reduce the harms associated with drug use during pregnancy.

Plan of This Book

Readers who are interested in how the PAD study was conducted may want to begin by reading appendix 1, "Women Talking to Women," where we describe our theoretical perspective and the methods we used to collect and interpret the study's data. In chapter 2, we set the stage for the rest of the analysis, presenting the demographics of the study population and a description of their lives, including their childhoods, drug-using patterns, relationships, and experiences of violence. Chapter 3 describes the difficult trajectory of drug-involved pregnancies: the discovery, the process of acceptance or termination, and the management of contradictory roles and significant others. In chapter 4, we delineate women's efforts to manage their pregnancies and reduce the potential harms of drug use during pregnancy.

Chapter 5 details the final showdown of birth and delivery, when months of ambivalence, fear, and harm-reduction efforts culminate in the glaring light of an institutional setting. In the final chapter, we address the question, "What should be done about pregnancy and drug use?"

Throughout these pages, you will hear the voices of Krista, Veronica, Sally, Marilyn, and all the other women who helped us to write this book. As you read, we want you to imagine the image of "mother" that looms over the shoulders of most American women. This imaginary mother-to-be is married to a committed father-to-be and plans her pregnancy carefully, eating nutritious foods and avoiding, at all costs, any unhealthy activities. Before she even conceives, she does everything she can to optimize her health. Once her children are born, she is an eternally nurturing and tireless woman who lives to care for her children and always makes the best choices for her family. This super mom is a mythical creature, of course, but she is a powerful presence in the minds of women who take on the demanding job of mothering in the waning years of the twentieth century.

You will learn about the poverty, violence, drug abuse, and sexual exploitation that characterized our interviewees' childhoods and how their unplanned pregnancies blurred the line between when their childhood ended and their womanhood began. Becoming pregnant under those conditions accelerated these women's loss of control over their bodies, their lives, and their futures. Yet everyone around them (themselves included) expected them to gain control over themselves and their drug use. Remember, this same mythical mother also loomed over these women's shoulders, but they attempted to meet her impossible challenges with severely constrained emotional, social, and material resources, usually at considerable personal cost.

2

Setting the

Stage

Life before
Pregnancy

Childhood was a difficult time for most PAD Project participants. For these women, the American dream—a nurturing family with two kids, two cars, and a house with a garden and a white picket fence—was, indeed, a distant dream. Nobody's family life matches this myth, but our interviewees' experiences were light years away. The women in our study grew up poor, lacking not only luxury goods but often the minimal necessities for normal life. Many were socially isolated. In dealing with the outside world, they commonly experienced embarrassment, insecurity, and shame.

Most interviewees grew up in disorganized and disrupted families. Single-parent households were common. Adult supervision was scarce, often because parents worked long hours at one or more jobs. Many women assumed adult responsibilities before they reached adolescence, regularly performing household tasks such as caring for younger children, cleaning, and cooking. Fifty-one percent of the women in our sample were under age eighteen when they had their first baby, becoming mothers before they themselves had had sufficient mothering. In telling their life stories, these women were unable to distinguish where childhood had ended and their womanhood began.

As young children, many had neither the encouragement nor the opportunity to do well in school because poverty, instability, and frequent relocations made regular attendance difficult. Problems at home interfered with schooling, and being bounced from school to school precluded establishing close ties with teachers or peers. The inner-city schools that study participants attended were usually underfunded, overcrowded, understaffed, and ill-equipped to deal with the girls' educational and emotional problems. About one-third of the women we interviewed dropped out of school before graduating. Fifty-eight percent eventually earned a high school diploma or its equivalent. None had received any specific job training, and only a few had ever been gainfully employed for more than a few months at a time.

Typically, study participants were exposed to drug use at a very young age. Often, they witnessed family members, friends, and neighbors using drugs; and by early adolescence most had begun to party with drugs themselves. Interviewees attributed their tendency to go wild during their teenage years to early family responsibilities that had left them little time for fun as children. Some women reported having been encouraged or forced to use drugs while being sexually assaulted in their homes.

Emotional, physical, and sexual abuse was an integral part of the childhoods of our interviewees. Seventy percent reported some sort of victimization, usually at the hands of male relatives or family friends. Women described going to bed fully clothed to impede fathers' access to their bodies during nightly visits. They recounted years of staying away from home after school to avoid being home alone with their mothers' untrustworthy boyfriends. Among these women's most vivid recollections of their childhoods were unwanted advances, unwanted touches, and fear.

For the women in our study, the world outside the family home was generally not much safer. Most were raised in neighborhoods plagued by gang warfare, crime, drug dealing, and violence. If there were churches and community organizations that might have helped these girls, they failed to do so. These young women fell through the cracks and landed on the streets, where their opportunities to obtain the American dream shrank with every passing year.

Becoming pregnant under these conditions accelerated women's loss of control over their bodies, their lives, and their futures. Yet as their pregnancies became public knowledge, they were expected to suddenly get control of themselves and quit using drugs altogether. In this chapter, we examine women's life experiences before getting pregnant in order to place their drug use into its social and psychological context. Their stories reveal how years of instability, insecurity, and violence conspired to deny them, first, the fundamental right to control their own bodies and, later, the right to mother their own children.

In this chapter, we set the stage, allowing our readers a look at interviewees' social worlds and experiences before becoming pregnant. By understanding the context of the women's drug use, we gain insight into the options available to this marginalized population. We can then begin to understand the importance of the mothering role in PAD participants' lives.

Demographic Description of the Study Population

One hundred and twenty pregnant and postpartum women were interviewed for this study. The majority (85 percent) were between twenty-two and thirty-five years old. The median age was twenty-nine. One-third were white, slightly more than half (52 percent) were African-American, and 7 percent were Latina. Three women were Pacific Islanders, and one was Creole.

Twenty-three percent of the women were Catholic, 12 percent mainstream Protestant (Methodist, Presbyterian, Lutheran, Episcopalian, or Unitarian), and 33 percent fundamentalist Protestant (Baptist, Pentecostal, or Seventh Day Adventist). Seven percent reported that they were spiritual but did not affiliate with any organized religion, and 15 percent said they were not religious. Two were black Muslims, and one was Jewish.

About half of the women grew up in working-class families, and 17 percent came from middle-class backgrounds. Thirty-six percent grew up in lower-class families in which their parents worked for menial wages or received public assistance.

Eighty percent of the study participants relied on public assistance at the time of the interview. Twelve percent of the women lived in publicly subsidized housing projects, 34 percent in apartments, and 21 percent in single room only (SRO) hotels rented either daily or weekly. The rest (33 percent) were homeless or living in shelters at the time of interview.

More than half (58 percent) of the interviewees had completed high school, with 10 percent completing some college. More than half (54 percent) had been convicted of misdemeanors, and 34 percent had been convicted of felonies. More than half had been in jail for five or more days, and 13 percent had served time in prison. Eighty-eight percent of the study participants had older children. Approximately 40 percent of these mothers had lost legal custodial rights, and 40 percent had relinquished children informally to family or friends.

Family Background

We asked, "Whom did you live with most of the time until you were sixteen?" Thirty-four percent reported living with single mothers, and 3 percent with single fathers. The remainder of the interviewees grew up in the homes of other relatives or foster parents. Sixteen percent were raised primarily by mothers and one or more stepfathers. During the course of their childhood, interviewees often lived in a series of settings: with other relatives, friends' families, foster care placements, juvenile detention facilities, or group homes. Some women felt they had been passed around from person to person, never having a real connection with any parental figure. Many of the women's childhoods were characterized by instability. Divorce, death, abandonment, violence, poverty, and substance abuse plagued these women's childhoods.

There were one or more detrimental relationships or conditions in about half (48 percent) of the women's families, such as parental addiction or severe emotional and sexual/physical abuse. Participants also suffered from neglect, abandonment, and consequent repeated foster care placement. One-half of the women left home by the time they were sixteen years of age, and 82 percent had left their homes by the time they were eighteen.

Instability

Divorce/Abandonment

In many cases, interviewees' mothers, like the study participants themselves, had sole responsibility for raising and supporting their children, which created enormous emotional and financial pressure. Parental divorce and abandonment were also sources of women's feelings of conflict and loss. Veronica, a thirty-four-year-old Latina, was raised in San Francisco's Mission District during the 1960s and 1970s. Her mother was left with eight children after her second marriage failed. Veronica and her sister raised their six brothers because their mother did not have the time, energy, or stability to do so.

Interviewer: So your mom and dad were together when you were growing up?

Veronica: They were until I was about six years old. And then my mom left my dad and she remarried. So then I had three stepbrothers from my mom's new husband. And then she divorced him and had two other kids. [At this point in the interview, Veronica began to cry.] So about that time, we were practically raising ourselves. It was rough.

Interviewer: God, you had a lot of responsibility when you grew up.

Veronica: Yeah, well, me and my sister, we practically raised my brothers because my mom couldn't do it. So me and her, we practically grew them up.

The responsibility for taking care of her younger siblings when she herself was just a child had profoundly negative consequences for Veronica. On the weekends, she and her sister would party hard to relieve the strain of their premature parental obligations. As she noted, "we didn't have much of a life ourself when we were young."

Another source of pain for Veronica and her siblings was

their mother's illness. When she became too ill to keep her children, she had to place Veronica and her siblings in foster care. Veronica began to cry again as she described the impact this had on all of them:

> It was hard for my brothers especially 'cause they were a lot younger. And right now, they go through a lot because of it. A lot of my brothers, they're not working. They kind of have a mixed-up life right now, too. A lot of them, like they'll smoke crack, which a couple of them are still on it. But it's hard for them, too. So I know what they go through.

Some single mothers looked to other family members to help raise their children. Alice, a thirty-two-year-old Filipina, who also grew up in San Francisco's Mission District, was raised by her uncle because her mother had to work two jobs:

> *Alice:* Mom was working. I had an uncle that my mom rented a room to, and he became a part of the family. And he took me over as, I guess, his adopted daughter. And he took me everywhere.
> *Interviewer:* How was your relationship?
> *Alice:* Beautiful. He took me from birth. He had children in the Philippines, so he couldn't see much of them. So he took me under his wing, and he just gave me everything. . . . And he loved me, and he did everything for me. If he was still around, I think a lot of things would be a lot easier.

Alice commented that although she had "a pretty nice childhood—no incest or abuse or anything," her father's abandonment left her with deep emotional scars:

> I'm learning now that rejection is the, pssss! It does a lot. I guess from my father not being around and being in the navy, and he remarried to another woman, 'cause

my mother didn't want him. So she rejected him. So it's just like it's gone down the line. And then any rejection I get from men or anybody. . . . I want to go use, or I want to go and do something that's abnormal, something to like run away and hide.

Death

The parent or parents of 16 percent of the participants died when the women were children. Parental deaths hurt women deeply and made them feel abandoned and alone. But in working-class and poor families, losing a parent also caused considerable financial strain for the remaining parent or extended family members. The women whose parents died often bounced from relative to relative. They felt like burdens to be put up with until they could be passed on to the next situation. Moving could also entail leaving other siblings, friends, and schools, and, in general, leaving the known for the unknown. For example, Lindley, a twenty-one-year-old African American, was six years old when her father died. Lindley was sent to live with her aunt and uncle. Life with them was very difficult:

> I understood why my mother had to leave, but I didn't understand my auntie 'cause she was real mean. And I didn't understand why she did the things she did to me. Yes, I guess I was supposed to have been perfect. So if I didn't do things like she wanted them done, if I didn't eat like she wanted me to eat or something like that, I'd get—I'd get whipped or something.

Unfortunately, things did not improve for Lindley even after she was reunited with her mother and her brothers when she was eight. Although the family was comfortable financially, there was a great deal of violence in the household. Her mother, who had been very affectionate when

Lindley was little, became physically abusive. Lindley thought her mother had changed as a result of the emotional strain of raising five young children alone after her husband's death.

Krista's mother died when she was eight years old. She had never known her father, and with her mother's death Krista and her half-brother became orphans. Reluctantly, her grandparents took in the two children. Krista felt they resented her half-brother, whose father was Korean. Her grandparents complained about having to take a "half-breed" into their home.

Krista returned to the topic of her mother's death while describing her current emotional state in another part of the interview: "Having a conversation like this [interview] would have been impossible for me to do before I reached this stage, 'cause even talking about my mother dying, I would get hysterically upset and just run out of the room in tears. And that was just two, three years ago."

Chandra, a forty-year-old white woman, whose adoptive mother died when she was five years old, described herself as a "latchkey kid." Her father worked until 8:00 P.M. during the weekdays and was rarely home. She did not get along with her stepmother, which created tension in the household. As a result, Chandra ran away to San Francisco's hippie scene when she was fourteen years old:

Chandra: And my mom died when I was five. She had cancer. He raised me himself.
Interviewer: Oh, my gosh. What was that like growing up?
Chandra: Really hard. Really hard. I was one of the original latchkey children.
Interviewer: For nine years you were with your dad without your mom?
Chandra: Yeah. And he worked from 6:00 in the morning until 8:00 at night. . . . And my father remarried,

and the woman he remarried, I didn't like her from the get-go. . . . One day, we had a fight in the house, and the next day she moved out, taking half the wedding picture. And after that, my father just fell apart, started beating me, started drinking. I couldn't take it. I left, no note, nothing.

Parental Substance Abuse

Some women associated their parents' drug and alcohol use with childhood problems. Veronica cried as she told the interviewer about her mother's substance use. Reflecting upon her own addiction to heroin and alcohol, she told us, "It's probably just like the same pattern, and I think it's going down from generation to generation."

Some of the abused women linked episodes of parental physical and sexual violence with drug or alcohol intoxication. Lola spoke at length about her alcoholic stepfather. When she was nine years old, he began forcing her to drink alcohol as it was easier to rape her when she was semiconscious. She finally reached the breaking point after years of abuse and shot him. Lola was placed in a mental hospital for four years. She still feels the pain of that abuse: "Bodily harm goes away after awhile. Emotional hurt leaves a scar for a long time, and you tend not to trust anybody." The trust violations that young girls experienced when fathers or father figures sexually assaulted them had consequences throughout women's adult lives.

Others claimed their parents' drinking and drug use were not related to family problems. Indeed, in some cases abusive parents were easier to manage when they were drunk or high because they would pass out rather than become violent. Parental drug and alcohol use, combined with unstable living conditions, made women feel unsafe, insecure, and unwanted. As children, their life situations were generally unpredictable and uncontrollable. They could not trust that their parents could or would protect them. This loss of control followed women into adulthood; many felt they had little control over their lives.

Lack of Parental Involvement

A two-parent household did not guarantee girls more financial or emotional stability. Both parents often had to work long hours for menial wages to support their families. Many of our interviewees believed that lack of parental involvement as a crucial missing piece of their childhoods.

Ethel, a twenty-nine-year-old Latina, was raised in the Bronx. Her father was a heroin addict who regularly beat her mother:

> My dad, he was a heroin user, and he was very abusive to my mom. And like it was a mental abuse on me and my brother. . . . But my mom didn't let him hit us. She would like put us in the closet or something so that when he was in his rage when there was no money or something for the drugs, he would just bang her up or just tear the house up or take the TVs and stereos and sell them and stuff.

Ethel's mother, who worked at McDonald's, was the sole financial provider for the family. Finances were tight, although she eventually was promoted to manager, which increased her income only slightly. When Ethel's father went to Vietnam, there was more stability in the house. When Ethel was fifteen years old, the family moved from a predominantly Puerto Rican neighborhood into a white community. She befriended white middle-class children whose lives took dramatically different paths:

And then at that time, I had a best friend who I met from the white community who, we're still friends today. She got married to her childhood sweetheart and moved out of the Bronx and she had her first baby. And that was nice. We went through that together and stuff, and it was like the kind of life that I would have wanted, you know, just to be happy and a marriage and have kids and to be a housewife. And it was just not possible for me.

A number of factors made conventional life seem inaccessible for Ethel: an abusive, addicted father; enduring racism; and having to drop out of school to help with family finances. The discordance between Ethel's idealization of the family lives in the white middle-class neighborhood and her own family life of abuse and poverty made her feel isolated and not at all like her girlfriend, who appeared to have a conventional, happy life-style. During Ethel's childhood, neither she nor her parents exercised any real control over their life circumstances, and nothing in her adult experience changed her sense of mastery.

Amy was a twenty-eight-year-old Latina whose parents were together during her childhood. They both worked long hours at night as janitors, and Amy rarely saw them. She was raised in San Francisco's Mission District in a neighborhood where drug use, delinquency, and crime were both prominent and alluring to a teenager with few other life options. Amy described moving around in the Mission:

There were a lot of things like [that] around here and stuff, like a lot of drugs going around and stuff. No matter where you moved to, it [drugs] was always there. Like say you tried to move from one neighborhood thinking you're gonna go to another one to get out of it, the same thing would be right there. I still live in the Mission. I moved from one side of the Mission to the other. But it's still the same. I think the best thing to do is maybe to—even if you moved out to somewhere else, I think that it would be the same thing there. It will always be around.

Even hard-working (if mostly absent) conventional parents could not protect Amy from the call of the streets. Long work hours kept parents out of the home and left children to fend for themselves in neighborhoods filled with drugs and crime.

Violence and Sexual Abuse

Many women grew up in families in which physical and sexual violence was prevalent. Seventy percent experienced emotional, physical, or sexual violence by family members, friends, and strangers. The women also witnessed violence in their homes or neighborhoods or had family members who were subjected to violence. Living with such violence was very debilitating. A number of the women recited lists of family members who had been killed. For example, Mariah's father had been shot in the head, her sister was shot in the heart by her boyfriend, an uncle had been killed in a car accident, and another uncle had been shot and paralyzed from the waist down. These litanies of loss were alarmingly common. It was a rare study participant who did not know someone, usually a relative, who had died a traumatic death. Again, lives soaked in violence and death gave birth to fatalistic notions characterized by the saying we heard over and over from the women: " when it's your time [to die], there ain't nothing you can do." How can you feel mastery and control over your own life situation when you never know when the phone is going to ring and yet another brother, cousin, or father has been killed? Or as several of the women put it, "you never know when the bullet with your name on it takes you out."

Regarding sexual violence, Donna talked about her stepfather, who began molesting her when she was nine years old:

> So he had me giving him head. I'm what—nine years old? And he's trying to get me to master this. And then he was gonna put it in me, his penis in me, but I was too small, and it's like he would have really messed me up. And he told me to put my fingers in myself every night to stretch it and stuff so he could do it. He wanted me to prepare, get ready.

Donna was twenty-two years old before she was able to tell her mother what her stepfather had done. She explained her feelings to us: "It's like, I guess as a kid I wanted her to see it without me telling her. It's like, 'You're my mother. You're supposed to see something's wrong.'"

Clinicians who work with incest survivors find that Donna's anger toward her mother is a common reaction to childhood sexual abuse. Incest survivors often blame their mothers for not protecting them. But the stepfather's abuse was not only a trust violation for Donna; it also ruined her relationship with her mother. Thus, sexual abuse increased Donna's sense of isolation and abandonment and taught her, and other participants' like her, that the world was a very unsafe place in which they had very little power or agency.

Bivette spent her childhood trying to help her mother discontinue drug use. Her mother and stepfather had frequent fights, which culminated in Bivette's mother shooting her stepfather. He survived the shooting but refused to press charges. Bivette moved out because she could not tolerate the situation any longer. The violence sickened her.

She told us: "I don't like being around violent things. I get really sick when I'm exposed to violence."

Amanda was another woman whose life was heavily affected by violence and sexual abuse. Her younger brother, who was blind, had a problem with bed wetting. One day her mother made him sit on a window ledge in their high-rise apartment building to punish him. He fell off the ledge and died after having his "head cracked open." For years, Amanda tormented herself for having failed to save her brother's life. She was also threatened by her stepfather, who began molesting her when she was ten years old. He raped her on a regular basis for five years, until she became pregnant. He had threatened her from the start, telling her, "If you ever tell anybody, I'll kill you. If you want to live to see twelve, you're not gonna say nothing."

When she became pregnant, she desperately wanted to keep the baby in order to have someone to love. Her stepfather, however, concocted a rape story and arranged for Amanda to have an abortion. As she reflected back on her life and the series of abusive men she had been involved with as an adult, Amanda said, "You know, I basically felt that God cursed me by bringing me into this world because everything I do—no matter what I do, life is just bad towards me."

Hillary's sad childhood sheds light on how living with the constant threat of violence affects a young woman's life. When Hillary was ten, her mother checked into the hospital to deliver Hillary's younger sister. At that point her stepfather began his ongoing efforts to sexually molest her. He drove her to a deserted part of town and threatened to leave her there if she did not have sex with him. For years, Hillary strategized to avoid being left alone with this man. She tried to rally her brother in her defense as well as invite friends to spend the night, hoping her stepfather would not have the nerve to molest her with another person in the room. Even when she was not being molested, she worried about it. Her worries and fears interfered with her schooling and sleep patterns: "Trying to go to school and you can't focus. And I wouldn't focus on school, no way, worried about what was going on at home. And wondering, 'Am I gonna be able to sleep tonight?'"

Sally's childhood was a nightmare. Both her parents abused her. She started running away from home at thirteen; but each time, even though she had visible bruises and scars on her body, the authorities would bring her back to her parents. When she was sixteen years old, she announced to her parents she was pregnant. Her mother and father threw her clothes out the front door onto the lawn. She never lived with them again.

Jessie was raised in San Francisco. Beginning when she was four years old, she was physically and sexually abused by her stepfather and then continuously sexually abused by a male baby-sitter. When she tried to tell her mother about the abuse from the baby-sitter, her mother would not listen. Jessie, however, does not blame her mother: "My mother, she didn't know. She was just working and trying to keep a roof over our heads." Her mother was also emotionally abusive, especially after Jessie's stepfather left.

Heather, a thirty-nine-year-old white woman, who grew up in Massachusetts with her seven brother and sisters, was raised by both her parents. Heather described her father as emotionally abusive toward her mother. This had a profound emotional impact on her in terms of how she felt about herself and toward men. She did not marry the father of her first child because she "did not want to be accused of trapping him into marriage, like her dad accused her mom." Heather also believed her father's drinking and gambling not only fueled his abuse but impoverished the family.

Violence for these women was not just perpetrated by family members. Many lived in a virtual reign of terror in neighborhoods with high rates of crime and violence. For example, Eliza, a twenty-nine-year-old African American, was raised in central Los Angeles, where violence was pervasive: "I was born and raised in central Los Angeles. My childhood there, I don't too much remember my childhood. But I do remember the neighborhood that I spent most of my memories in, the schools and some of friends and witnessed a lot of murders and gang beatings."

Lindley was raised with four brothers by an abusive mother. She described herself as a timid person, afraid of everyone and everything when she was young. When she began attending high school, she realized that showing fear in the ghetto was a serious liability. Her brothers, who did a lot of fighting themselves, encouraged her to stand up for herself, saying, "don't let nobody hit you." They taught her how to fight, act tough, and protect herself. She worried that her independence and smart mouth would get her into trouble but conceded that while she was living in a violent world, it behooved her to react in a tough and violent manner.

The neighborhoods that the poorest participants grew up in were, in many instances, veritable combat zones. Between gang warfare, police raids, random shootings, and drug dealing, fear became a way of life. Our findings concur with other studies that link childhood experiences of violence, sexual abuse, and physical abuse with the increased likelihood that a woman will develop drug and alcohol problems later in life (Reed 1991). For many of our study participants, drug use was a way of numbing themselves from fear of ambient violence and emotional pain caused by lost family members, lost trust and security, and ultimately lost childhoods.

Exceptional Families

Some women reported that their family lives had been happy and their parents supportive. Emily, a thirty-two-year-old white woman, was raised in the San Francisco Bay area. Her parents were happily married and worked throughout Emily's childhood. She told her interviewer: "They are still married to this day, and they still have the same house they moved into when I was four years old. They were good parents. Couldn't ask to come from any better stock or anything. My dad was the salt of the earth. Went to work to support the family."

Similarly, Kelly, a thirty-five-year-old African American, described her childhood as very stable. Her parents were supportive and financially secure. Several members of her family, including Kelly, had college degrees and owned their own homes. Kelly expressed her proud feelings for her mother throughout the interview:

> My moms is this totally straight person, this southern Christian woman. She never drinks, never smokes. My moms worked eight days a week. She's seventy years old now, and you would not believe it. She was vegetarian before being a vegetarian was cool. My mother is just perfect. If I could just be half the person my moms is.

Although these women were spared the chaotic childhoods so characteristic of most of our study participants, their pleasant memories inflicted their own brand of pain. Emily and Kelly experienced their drug use as a great source of shame, informing us that their parents did not deserve to have such rotten kids. Mindy described her mother's anguish: "I'd be in the room, and I would hear her crying. And I knew why she was crying. So I'd just cover my head with the pillow, and I would cry, too, 'cause I hated to hear her cry. It seems like I was always doing something to make her cry."

Education

For many study participants, education was a low priority. Furthermore, poverty, general instability, violence, drugs, unemployment, and boredom made concentration on schoolwork extremely difficult.

As we detailed previously, Veronica's childhood was very unstable. Her mother married and divorced several times and had a total of eight children. During her early years, Veronica moved frequently and transferred among schools regularly. This caused her to fall behind; she ended up in a continuation high school and finally dropped out altogether in her second-to-last year:

> School, I liked school. It was okay. But we were mostly moving around a lot. My mom was always moving from place to place. Like I said, when we were younger, she had left us with our dad, just me and my sister and my brother. Well, she went off and got married. And then we were going from school, and then when she'd come back and get us, we'd transfer to another school. And that's mostly what it was. She was always moving, always. And I went up to the eleventh grade, and it was like in a continuation school, my high school. But junior high school was more steadier than high school. And that's as far as I went in high school. It was okay. It was okay. But I had gotten pregnant, so I dropped out. So that's where that started. So that was the end of my schooling.

The poor quality of the schools themselves contributed to the school dropout rate (42 percent). The women complained of underfunded, overcrowded, and dilapidated educational facilities. Krista called the school she attended in a southern California school district "a joke":

> School, the school system was incredible. I mean, I never went, and they kept pushing me. You know, I was one of those kids that was just pushed through grade by grade by grade. Eleventh grade or whatever was when I finally dropped out completely, but I never even went. It was ridiculous. Luckily, I'm lucky to have learnt to know how to read and write . . . and I basically learned that when my mother was alive. Seriously. Because I was just pushed through the system, and it was ridiculous. I mean, I wasn't gonna graduate, you know, with the credits I had, but on paper it looks good. I was on eleventh grade, and I was this many years old. It was crazy. Get me out of that school system as fast as it can with the rest of the kids, like herd them through.

Krista dropped out of school when she was seventeen, shortly after she had her first child.

At fourteen, Emily became a full-time waitress. That same year, she began to use stimulant drugs in an attempt to control her weight. Soon she was cutting classes. But instead of putting Emily in a special program, the high school expelled her.

Interviewer: So, now, did you finish high school?
    Emily: No. . . . This school just wrote me a letter and just said, "Well, we got plenty of people who are waiting to be here, so please don't come back in January." So, that's how. . . .
Interviewer: So, you said . . . ?
    Emily: Okay, I guess [laughs]. Actually, I thought it was kind of a shame because that semester I was tak-

ing driver's ed., and I was just starting, just No-
vember, I was starting to attend a little bit better
and wanting to come to school. By that time, it
was almost too late.

Poverty and general instability made it difficult for many
study participants to attend school regularly. In addition to
these disruptive factors, some women claimed that their
main reason for leaving school was the lure of street life
and drug use. For these women, drug use and the consequent life-style either decreased their school attendance or
kept them from going to school at all.

We have mentioned that Amy had little parental supervision while she was growing up. By the time she got to
high school, hanging out with her friends and drinking beer
in the park was much more interesting than sitting in bor-
ing, overcrowded classrooms. By her junior year, Amy was
cutting more classes than she was attending, and she decided to drop out:

Interviewer: So when did you quit high school?
      Amy: When I was in eleventh grade.
Interviewer: And what do you remember about that? Did you
             start working?
      Amy: No, I just stopped going. Like I started cutting
             too much and stuff. Then I just stopped going.
Interviewer: So what was going on instead? You were cutting
             school and . . . ?
      Amy: Drinking and smoking weed all the time. Smok-
             ing, smoking weed.

Other women used drugs but managed to stay in school.
For example, Naomi, a twenty-nine-year-old white woman,
had an unconventional childhood. Her mother was an art-
ist, and her father taught history. Both were Christian Scientists, and there were no drugs of any sort in the house.
When Naomi was ten years old, her family toured Europe

in a van. She went to school there for six months but never finished eighth grade. She was very bright, however; and when her family returned to the United States, Naomi was placed in advanced placement courses in high school. These classes exposed her to young people far wealthier than she and also introduced her to the world of drugs:

> *Naomi:* So I got sent to this "better" school, which was actually rich kids, and we were more like working-class kinda people. Everybody was like freaked out. There was a hell of a lot of drugs there.
>
> *Interviewer:* Were there more drugs there than . . . ?
>
> *Naomi:* All the drugs, yeah. There was more——people that are so rich, they all seem to have problems.

Naomi described the high levels of drug use as well as the fact that the school was lacking academically:

> I started cutting classes, not really wanting to be there, and having fun and running away and going to the beach or going to Hollywood, going here and going there. It was a joke, and the teachers were a joke. I can think of a few good teachers I had. L.A. city schools are the worst. They are the worst. They just kind of encourage you to be a juvenile delinquent. They don't care. I graduated, actually, with honors from my school, and I was never there. It was a joke.

A number of women claimed drug use as their primary reason for leaving school. It appears, however, that drug use was just one of many factors that may have made school attendance problematic, including abusive parents, frequent moves, and emotional trauma.

Several gender-specific problems or conditions interfered with the women's educational options. These included differential accountability for pregnancy, child care, and housework. *Child care* in this instance refers to the care of younger siblings as well as one's own children.

After her first sexual experience, Rhonda became pregnant at sixteen years old and decided to keep the baby. School officials pressured her to stop attending her regular high school and transfer to a "pregnancy school," but Rhonda insisted on completing her senior year and graduating with her class. Rhonda was proud to be pregnant, and she loved being showered with attention. After her child was born, however, her mother stepped in to care for her infant daughter, and Rhonda reentered the party circuit.

In contrast to Rhonda's situation, other young women found the responsibility of caring for a baby overwhelming and high school graduation impossible. Jenny was raped and became pregnant when she was fifteen years old. The emotional trauma of the rape and the physical toll of her pregnancy caused her to drop out of school during her junior year.

Additionally, the gendered division of household labor frequently meant that the young women had to assume responsibility for housework, which curtailed the time available for schoolwork. Evania, a thirty-three-year-old Latina, spoke with some bitterness about this during her interview: "Well, my mom used to work and stuff, so I had to take care of the kids. Well, I was the girl, right? So I had to wash the dishes and cook and stuff, and watch my little brother and sister, 'cause my older brothers—they were too busy messing up [getting into trouble], right?"

Similarly, Ethel detailed the obstacles to her academic success. In junior high school, she fell behind when her mother kept her home to baby-sit her younger siblings. When it came time for high school, her poor attendance record left her with a limited range of options. Despite being a good student, Ethel was relegated to a vocational school, which she found uninspiring:

> My mom kept me out of school and stuff. And I was a pretty good student. I had good grades and stuff. I graduated out of junior high as an ESP [gifted] student. And then, because of my attendance, I didn't have a wide choice of schools that I could go to. So I went to vocational school. And it was like a total hang out. Then I hooked up with this girl named J., and she taught me how to smoke cigarettes and smoke pot and drink beer. And so that's what I did for three years. I was still in ninth grade for like three years. It's not like I had a learning problem. It was just so much dysfunction in my family that, you know—and the crowd I chose to hang out with. So I didn't even go to school.

Ethel was eventually placed in a program for troubled youth, which she said was wonderful. She finally felt she was being taught something useful and interesting. With the assistance of this program, she was able to graduate from high school. Ethel then began business school, where she studied computer science. She said, "I did real good. Again, I was on the dean's list. I was a good student."

Unfortunately, once again Ethel's plans were disrupted by family violence. Her brother shot and killed a policeman's daughter, and Ethel witnessed the crime. People in their neighborhood began talking badly about her family and taunting Ethel about her brother. The combination of grief and shame prompted her family to move, and once again Ethel was forced to quit school—this time for good.

Responsibility for one's own children or siblings and housekeeping tasks were differentially assigned to girls. Consequently, in addition to the normal challenges of adolescence, these women were frequently juggling parental obligations when they were still children themselves. Pregnancy, poverty, and abuse contributed to their lack of education and preparation for the time when they would enter work worlds and attempt to be in control of their own lives.

Early Drug Use

Most study participants started using drugs early and became regular users by the time they were seventeen years old. Most (90 percent) had smoked marijuana, 50 percent had used heroin, 78 percent had either smoked or injected powder cocaine, and 30 percent had used methamphetamines. Interviewees also used legal drugs. Thirty-five percent reported they currently drank alcohol, and 54 percent said they drank during pregnancy. Eighty-one percent reported smoking tobacco, and 86 percent had smoked during pregnancy. Our interviewees, like their middle-class counterparts, began using drugs to satisfy curiosity, to take risks, to alleviate boredom, to experience specific drug effects for recreation or for self-medication. Study participants often cited psychological problems, depression, anxiety, or low self-esteem as important factors in pushing them into abusive drug-using patterns.

Chandra's parents bought her in a black market adoption. She started using heroin when she was fourteen years old, after running away to be a California hippie. Her biological mother was a heroin addict; and this, she felt, accounted for her early physiological problems and later addiction to heroin. During her childhood, she was plagued with chronic health problems:

> So they adopted me, and they couldn't figure out why
> I was always fussy. I was always crying. Until the time
> I was seven years old, if I got up too fast, I would walk

into the kitchen and fall down and just pass out. And my father knew at that point [that her biological mother had been a heroin addict], but he wouldn't tell the doctors. The doctors kept giving me iron thinking it was anemia. And my whole memory of life is not having any energy except for hyperactive energy.

The first time Chandra used heroin she found relief for her chronic fatigue:

> *Chandra:* So I came up to San Francisco, and I met some people. And they said, "Have you ever done any smack?" And I said, "Oh, yeah. Sure." Of course, I had not.
>
> *Interviewer:* Did you know what it was?
>
> *Chandra:* No, I didn't. They said, "Well, how often do you do it?" I said, "Oh, two or three times a week." So they gave me a shot that probably should have killed a horse. They had robbed the Haight Street pharmacy for some liquid pharmaceutical opium. Everybody else nodded out. And I did the shot, fell back for maybe forty-five seconds. I then got up, made a spaghetti dinner, cleaned the house, ironed the clothes for the people, scrubbed the bathroom floor. For the first time in my life, I had energy. And I went, "Why are people saying heroin is bad?". . . And at that point, I said, "This is what I want to do for the rest of my life. Why is it illegal?"

At about the same time Chandra found the drug that gave her much-needed energy, her father abandoned her. She started socializing almost exclusively with drug users, and she quit school, thereby limiting her future employment opportunities.

Jessie, who was sexually abused by her baby-sitter at four years old, starting taking her mother's Valium to offset her depression. Her use escalated during adolescence. When memories of this abuse emerged in adulthood, she went on an extended crack binge.

Veronica was surrounded by drug use while growing up. When she was seven years old, she watched her uncle inject heroin:

> Oh, you know, all my uncles, they were all drug users. And I can remember at the age of seven, six years old, my uncles—they used to live with my mom—and I had three of them that were drug abusers, right? And my favorite uncle, I remember, I think I must have been about six or seven the first time he walks into my mom's house, he runs in—and he used to be a burglar, right? He used to break into people's house[s], and I always remember him coming to my mom with a handkerchief full of jewelry. And I never thought nothing about it until one day I was home by myself and nobody was there. My uncle comes running in. He didn't care. He put his foot up on the chair and alls I seen him do was stick out his syringe and start shooting hisself up, right? And from that day on, I have never forgotten that day. So I always used to tell myself, "God, I'm never gonna do that, never." And to this day, I still think about it. I say, "God, how can I do it after what I've seen my uncle . . . ?" And plus, my other uncles going through it, in and out of prison all their life.

When she was thirteen, Veronica started drinking with friends. Two years later, after her boyfriend introduced her to them, she snorted and injected heroin and cocaine. Veronica recalled that injecting heroin made her feel "really mellow, really relaxed." After she had her first child at eighteen, she started using daily.

Veronica thought she got into drug use because her childhood was such a nightmare:

> *Veronica:* Well, I grew up here in San Francisco. . . . And it
> wasn't a very good childhood.
> *Interviewer:* Why do you say that?
> *Veronica:* Well, I don't know. I just hate to get into it. It's
> real emotional, my childhood. [She begins to cry.]
> So every time I think about it, it's fucked. I think
> that's why a lot of times I got into drugs, because
> of my mom and my dad.

Emily, whose family was very stable when she was growing up, started smoking marijuana at fourteen years old because she got in with the wrong crowd. Before she turned
sixteen, she began injecting speed. Initially, she used speed
for weight control and because it made her feel "exuberant." A year later, she met an older (thirty-six-year-old) man,
who encouraged her to escalate her use. Later on, this man
forced her at gunpoint to shoot speed, and eventually she
ended up in the hospital for an overdose.

When Krista was nine years old, her mother died, and
she began smoking marijuana. She remembers one incident
very vividly:

> I was nine years old, and this girl was sixteen years old
> and she asked me to smoke some pot which I thought
> was really just pot. And we were up at the fort, you
> know, this little thing in the field. And I smoked this
> thing I thought was just pot and it wasn't. I didn't know
> what it was at the time. I had no idea what was wrong
> with me. I was really . . . something was wrong. A few
> years later, when I tried PCP . . . I realized what it was,
> okay? . . . I was nine years old, and this girl, she just
> simply didn't want to get high by herself. And she didn't
> tell me what she was giving me. She thought it was
> funny or something.

When Krista was sixteen, she met her children's father,

who introduced her to cocaine and heroin use. Previously, she had tried a number of drugs, including amphetamines, LSD, and hashish. Cocaine was the first drug she injected. Soon after, she was shooting heroin as well. She felt that the relationship with her children's father revolved around drug use: "That's basically what our relationship was, being high." Krista believed that loneliness and depression precipitated her drug use. On a speed binge the summer before the interview, she remembered that when she was sixteen she had been raped by the Huntington Beach police while being arrested. She realized then this was a source of her lifelong psychological pain:

> See, I had always remembered getting drunk that night and getting arrested. But I didn't remember being raped. And I remember now. I remember waking up at home beat up. Two black eyes, a concussion, broken ribs. I mean, I remember that 'cause I was beat up for weeks. . . . Okay, now, like I can remember those things, and it's made me feel like I know now why I've been sad a lot. I don't feel like that anymore, you know? I mean, being sad a lot was why, and lonely, feeling lonely, is a lot of the reason why I want to be high.

Like all of our other interviewees, Krista had a number of factors that contributed to her early drug abuse: her mother's death when she was eight years old; growing up with strict and unsympathetic grandparents; dropping out of an overcrowded and indifferent high school; being introduced to PCP before she was ten; and, at sixteen, getting pregnant by a dangerously abusive man, who introduced her to cocaine and heroin injection. The rape was one more horrifying event in this sad but typical life story.

Licit and Illicit Work and Welfare

As we mentioned earlier in this chapter, 80 percent of the study participants were receiving some type of public assistance. Only six women were employed; four were receiving unemployment benefits, and nineteen relied entirely on illegal activities for support. Interviewees' median income was $650 per month, and they were supporting an average of one other person.

With few exceptions, interviewees had limited conventional work experience. Some had rarely or never been legally employed. Women with licit work experience held menial jobs at minimum wage levels. The combination of poor pay and expensive child care was defeating. The interviewees who had custody of their older children usually had primary responsibility for their children. Consequently, costly or inaccessible child care complicated their work lives or kept them out of the workplace and dependent on Aid to Families with Dependent Children (AFDC). Women on all types of public entitlement programs (such as General Assistance or Social Security Insurance) occasionally performed legal jobs under the table. They risked criminal penalties and heavy fines to supplement meager welfare allotments.

Expensive drug use and subsistence income propelled women into illegal work careers, primarily shoplifting, sex work, and drug sales. Evania "boosted" to generate income. She and her friend would first stop at their neighborhood drug store and smuggle out a bundle of paid stickers from behind the counter. From there, they headed for Safeway:

> We'd take them little stickers into Safeway and just stick them on Safeway's Pampers. And then when you go up to the counter, they'd say, "And these Pampers,

too." We'd say, "Oh no, I got these at Walgreens." So you go to Safeway and get your WIC [publicly funded food program for women and children] shit, you know, your eggs and your milk and stuff, and while you're doing that you pick up Pampers. And every time I'd go through, I'd take about four bags of Pampers. And I'd go to Safeway every day. So the Pampers I wasn't using, I was selling to my neighbors. Everybody knew me as the Pampers lady. They'd come and tell me what size they needed. I supplied the whole territory.

Other women, like Ethel, earned money or drugs from prostitution—or, as they called it, "dating." Ethel said: "I was fucking and doing everything. And I got to the point where, just for example, I fucked somebody for three dollars, man, 'cause I was really hungry and I had spent all my money."

Rhonda exchanged sex for money: "I was a prostitute and if I did—well, I don't know if you would really call it prostitute, but it was with people that liked me. Like maybe two or three peoples. But from what I can recollect, they were like boyfriends. But they were like older men, and they would try to mess with me."

Later in her interview, Rhonda talked about the rules she had set for herself regarding this work:

I did not get high with men. I'd get high with my cousins and stuff. A man can have a pocketful of drugs. He couldn't lure me nowhere and get me high. If we gonna take care of business, we gonna take care of business. You give me my money, I'll go buy my own drugs. No, I don't want to sit up and do nothing with you for drugs. If it wasn't for money, it wasn't at all. Damn! You gonna wake up, you gonna sit up there and smoke, and then you're gonna sell your body? Wake up and don't have nothing? You might wake up hungry. You know, you do wake up hungry.

Many of the women interviewed for the PAD Project came from poor, unstable, often abusive homes. As they shared their childhood experiences, what stood out were the challenges these women faced even before their own drug use became a problem. With few exceptions, the troubled trajectory characterizing these women's lives had its origin in painful family histories that severely wounded the young girls who matured into the women we interviewed. These women lived painful lives characterized by truncated childhoods, drug abuse, violence, poverty, racism, and demeaning work. The women did not have control over basic things such as who touched their bodies. Within this context of social stigma and personal chaos they discovered their pregnancies.

3

The Troubled

Trajectory of

Pregnancy

For a variety of reasons—primarily their lack of a sense of control over their futures—most women in this study did not practice birth control. Not only was their status as addicts built around the idea that they had lost control of their drug use, but their early life experiences, particularly experiences of sexual exploitation and sexual violence, had prevented them from developing a self-concept that included personal agency. In addition, many women believed that they could not get pregnant, a belief reinforced by the fact that their drug use often disrupted their menstrual cycles.

Unplanned Pregnancies

Even under the best of circumstances, women find it difficult to successfully manage contraception. As women of childbearing age, PAD staff members understood the complexities of coordinating sexuality, romantic relationships, and birth control technologies. For the majority of the women in this study, successful family planning was not a feasible option. Most of their pregnancies came as a complete surprise. Most (112) decided to have their babies. Right from the start, interviewees understood the inherent conflict between the drug-using world they lived in and the social role their pregnancies conferred upon them. By continuing the pregnancy, they began the difficult process of trying to integrate the roles of drug user and mother.

Sexual Violence and the Lack of Control

PAD Project women, whose lives were marked by poverty, neglect, exploitation, and violence, had never felt in control of any part of their lives, including their own bodies. Typically their introduction to sexuality occurred during childhood, often via molestation or rape by male relatives or other older males living in their household. As a result, in a very concrete way, women learned early that their bodies were not theirs to control. These experiences of violent sexual exploitation made it difficult for women to later exert control over their adult sexual relations and had obvious implications for adult contraceptive use.

Heather described a scene that unfortunately had been typical in her life:

> We had a fight one evening. He had his own little apartment, and I was still at home. We had two dogs, and his puppy chewed up his underwear and sandals. I said, "Just don't leave your stuff hanging around so that the puppy will get at it like that." Well, we happened to be at his place one night, and that was when the puppy had chewed a special-made pair of his sandals. He kicked the puppy out the door. I mean, he busted its

hip. I just went off and said, "You crude, heartless bastard. I'm leaving." He chased me all the way up the hill. I was running home, and he dragged me back down. And that's when we had our sex. And I swear that's the night I got pregnant.

Lucy, who had a long history of abusive relationships, was asked what she did when the men in her life became violent:

I have to do whatever they want me to do. That's why I have trouble making decisions now, because I'd rather just say—forget it, and go on and do it [have sex] and cut all that out than to have a man jumping on me all the time. I'm not a violent-type person, and I don't like pain. So I just do it. Just like my father. My father done stomped me and beat me.

Our findings are consistent with other research that indicates high levels of past and present exploitation and violence among pregnant drug users (Fagan 1995; Miller, Downs, and Testa 1989; Reed 1991; Regan, O'Malley, and Finnegan 1982). Overall, 70 percent of the interviewees reported they had been in one or more relationships in which they were physically battered by a male partner. Of the eighty-four women who had been assaulted by their partners, thirty-eight (45 percent) reported being battered during their current or most recent pregnancy. Thirty percent (twenty-five) were in an abusive relationship at the time of their interview.

In her influential article "Sexual Decision-Making and AIDS: Why Condom Promotion among Vulnerable Women Is Likely to Fail," Dooley Worth (1989) discusses the manner in which incest, economic hardship, physical abuse, and cultural influences shape women's use of contraceptive

technologies. She emphasizes the middle-class bias underlying the concepts of family planning and consistent birth
control use. These approaches assume the existence of sexual
equality between men and women as well as women's faith
in their abilities to exercise meaningful control over their
lives. Dorothy Roberts, in her historic treatise about the
ongoing assault on African-American women's reproductive
liberty, makes an equally powerful case regarding the racist
nature of American reproductive policies. Roberts (1997)
argues persuasively that African-American women are jus-
tifiably suspect of white society's attempt to curtail their
reproduction. Our interviewees' accounts of their lives echoed
both Roberts's and Worth's theses regarding the relationship between women's past experiences and their influence
on current birth control use.

Women in this study not only found it problematic to
engage in long-range family planning; they also found it difficult to negotiate with male partners regarding condom use.
Impoverished women with expensive drug habits who engaged in commercial sexual activities with strangers feared
that insisting on a condom might cause them to lose a cus-
tomer. In committed relationships, asking for condom use
could be interpreted by the partner as evidence of her infidelity or evidence that she suspected her male partner of
infidelity. In volatile relationships, women worried that even
discussing condom use would trigger violent responses.

Drug Use

Another contributing factor to the sporadic use of
birth control was the impact of extended drug use on
women's bodies. For many women, the combination of long-
term drug use and erratic eating habits resulted in men-
struation cessation. In addition to the loss of appetite

induced by stimulant drug use, many women were malnour-
ished due to limited financial resources strained even further
by expensive drug habits. Several of our older interviewees
reported they had not menstruated in years. Lorraine, who
was thirty-eight years old, explained, "I thought maybe
because of all those years of using drugs, I couldn't get pregnant again." Some women believed the drugs' pharmaco-
logical actions contributed to infertility.

In addition to the irregular menses that led some women
to believe they could not conceive, many attributed morning sickness to drug withdrawal. Thus, the general level of
nausea that accompanied coming down from drug highs
masked pregnancy symptoms. Liz was using heroin daily
when we interviewed her. She became pregnant for the first
time when she was nineteen years old. Liz did not have an
abortion until she was twenty-five weeks along because she
did not know she was pregnant. In retrospect, she realized
one indicator of pregnancy was that she was vomiting daily
instead of only once a week: "When you're addicted to
heroin, you don't have your period, right? You don't have
your menstrual period. So you don't know you're pregnant.
And you throw up a lot anyways because this drug makes
you throw up, right? So I had no idea I was pregnant, and I
was in my sixth month of pregnancy."

Liz had her third abortion three weeks before our interview. As she discussed her abortions, she said that she believed terminating the pregnancies was the right thing for
her to do. She explained, "I don't think women who are
addicted to drugs should have babies anyway."

Methods of Discovery

There were a number of ways in which women discovered they were pregnant. Some recognized their symptoms

quickly, particularly if they had been pregnant before. Lindley recalled:

> When I missed it [her period] two times—I went, "Wait a minute." And that really tripped me out because it was like the third week of my pregnancy [when] I felt like I was pregnant, but I was like, " . . . Well, I can't get pregnant. I'm not pregnant." But then four or five weeks come, and I'm throwing up and hating this guy for nothing. "Just get away from me." Crying because I can't get pickles. I'm like, "God, I know I'm not pregnant." But then I thought, "Maybe I am."

Jackie purchased an over-the-counter pregnancy test to confirm her suspicions:

> I took pregnancy tests, but they kept coming up negative. But I think what it was, I had so much dope in my system my tests were coming up wrong. And then when I found out I was pregnant with him, I was already four months. [Before that] I was, "Well, I can keep using cause I'm not hurting him. There's nothing there." So, I mean, I ain't hurting nobody but myself. So I went on ahead.

These early detection situations were infrequent. Most women discovered/acknowledged pregnancy after abortion was no longer a feasible (for legal or personal reasons) option. Drug use not only disrupted the women's menstrual cycles but interfered with their ability to diagnose pregnancy.

For example, when we interviewed Vicky, she was thirteen weeks' pregnant with her second child. When asked how she found out she was pregnant, she commented, "Heroin hides stuff, like pregnancy." It was her partner, however, who noticed that her nipples looked different and wanted her to go in for a breast examination. During her interview Vicky remembered, "If it wasn't for the test saying I'm pregnant, I wouldn't know I'm pregnant."

Nelly, an African American in her mid-thirties, had eight-month-old twin boys. She had a long history of drug use, dealing, prostitution, and shoplifting but had been trying to discontinue drug use since the birth of her boys. When asked how she first realized she was pregnant, Nelly replied: "A couple of people had looked at me, and they didn't know me from Adam, and they was talking about, 'Oh, you're so pretty pregnant.' [And she replied,] 'I'm not pregnant. You're crazy.' Then I threw up one morning, and I thought, where did this come from?"

Mindy was the furthest along without discovery:

Interviewer: When did you first realize you were pregnant?
Mindy: [seven months' pregnant] Oh, just last week. I looked down—I mean, I just couldn't believe it.

As these quotations illustrate, few women planned to become pregnant. Some believed they were incapable of conceiving. Often pregnancy came as a shock.

Like other women of childbearing age, interviewees went back and forth thinking maybe they could be pregnant or maybe their morning nausea was just normal indigestion. This self-diagnosing process was further influenced by women's social contexts and their readiness or reticence to mother. In short, discovery of pregnancy is for many women a very complicated social psychological process. For women who use drugs these complications are compounded by fears concerning the possible effects of their drug use on forming fetuses and their own and almost everybody else's expectations that they must immediately implement life-style changes, particularly cessation of all drug use. Given the difficulties of discontinuing often lifelong drug-using patterns and setting in motion life-style changes with limited social and economic resources, Mindy's surprise at looking down and finding herself seven months' pregnant becomes easier to comprehend.

Responses to Discovery

Regardless of how they learned they were pregnant, once pregnancy was discovered, many women confronted a difficult set of decisions. They immediately weighed the possible impact of past drug use on the fetus. The pregnant drug user needed to admit to herself and others (fathers, families, friends, health care providers, and social workers) that her growing fetus was being exposed to drugs.

From the women's perspective, even if they quit using or significantly reduced their use, their baby-to-be could still be at serious risk. Additionally, if the women accepted the pregnancy but continued to use drugs, they became members of a group even more marginalized and stigmatized than women drug users—*pregnant* drug users. Most interviewees endured guilt-ridden periods of debate and uncertainty.

Study participants' responses to pregnancy varied. Most, however, were cloaked with ambivalence. Even before they were certain they were pregnant, most women began to consider what had already happened since conception. They examined their current living situations and relationships with the fathers-to-be and decided to terminate or continue the pregnancy. Unlike other newly pregnant women, however, our interviewees had a reflective process that was much more ambivalent. On the one hand, fetal drug exposure and the need to discontinue drug use pushed women to consider abortion. But at times the women's drug use meant that they discovered the pregnancy late or were unable to get to an abortion clinic. Then they were forced to accept the pregnancy.

For some women, acknowledging that they were pregnant was very difficult. Naomi used both speed (methamphetamine) and heroin and had miscarried two weeks before her interview. She wanted to miscarry, so she used medicinal teas and detoxified from drugs cold turkey. Naomi explained how she realized she was pregnant: "I was like crying and acting weird and waking up in the middle of the night. Like I said, I was never pregnant. I've never used birth control in my life. And I never got pregnant."

Upon confirmation of her pregnancy, she felt "incredible fear. It seems weird that something that should bring you a lot of joy and happiness is—that it's my worst fear. That's the only thing I'm afraid of is being pregnant. It scares me to death because then I have to make a decision. Like, what do I do, you know? And I know that I cannot possibly, I just cannot go around having babies."

Nancy's narrative exemplifies many women's concerns regarding drug-exposed pregnancies. Worried, she told us, "Look, I've shot speed. I've shot heroin, and I'm afraid I'm going to have a baby with very bad problems." Women who used crack had more worries than the speed and heroin users did. We hypothesize that the hysteria generated in the media about crack babies during the time we conducted the interviews contributed significantly to crack-using participants' anxieties. Christine, like other interviewees, began to see her unborn fetus as a potential "drug baby" too damaged to be allowed to be born:

> That's what makes me think I don't need this baby, 'cause I'm using. I like drugs. I know they're no good for me. I know what they do to my life. But right now, this is where I want to be. I've got a doctor's appointment tomorrow [to discuss an abortion] because this is being stupid. Why bring these drug babies into the world like that?

Not all women were unhappy to discover they were pregnant. For those women who had assumed they were infertile, pregnancy was cause for great joy, living proof their drug use had not impaired their reproductive capacities. These women viewed their pregnancies as opportunities to change their life-styles, almost as if the pregnancy was a special gift to provide them with new hope and resolve.

Christy was delighted to learn she was four months' pregnant. She had worried that several abortions and heavy drug use had rendered her unable to conceive. During this pregnancy, she prostituted only occasionally to support herself, sucking her stomach in and wearing loose clothing.

Kristen, a twenty-two-year-old African American, was fifteen weeks' pregnant. Since discovering her pregnancy a week before the interview, she had quit smoking crack, cut out coffee, and stopped turning tricks. She hoped this baby would make up for all the experiences she missed with her first daughter. Kristen and women like her saw their pregnancies as a source of new hope, another (or first) chance to become a good mother and to make up for past transgressions.

The Role of Partners

In addition to their own feelings about their pregnancies, the women had to negotiate or attempt to avoid partners' reactions. Some women chose to conceal their pregnancies from the babies' fathers. Those women who chose to conceal or terminate the pregnancy did not want to deepen or sometimes even continue the relationship with these men. Jenny articulated women's rationales for keeping abusive and controlling daddies in the dark: "I'm not fixing to have this baby. This is a very abusive relationship. I'm not going to have him all deep in my ass by having his baby."

Similarly, Darleen was uncertain whether or not she wanted to stay with her partner. She knew that acknowledging his paternity would make him feel he had the right to control her actions. After she informed him, he continually threatened to hit her in the stomach if she did not submit to his demands. Darleen lamented, "I know I'm not gonna take too much more hitting."

Another study participant, who had been homeless for a year, detailed her initial reaction to learning she was pregnant: "I said, 'No, God would not do this to me. We don't have any way to live.' I started filling in, my chest, my dress—and getting hungry and bitchy if he [her partner] didn't let me to go the [soup kitchen] to eat. He kept yelling, 'All you think about is eating! Eating! You must be pregnant, you bitch!'"

Disclosing their pregnancies was fraught with danger for women with controlling and abusive partners. Several women chose to keep silent and terminate. Other women informed the fathers-to-be and found that "having their babies" made them more vulnerable to the men's demands and restrictions. In these types of relationships, the male partner's sense of ownership of the baby expanded his sense of entitlement to ownership of the woman herself. The women found their men to be "deeper in their ass" than ever before.

Other Significant Others' Reactions

In addition to their partners, most women had to consider the reaction of the other significant people in their lives. Cheryll, a thirty-seven-year-old white heroin, cocaine, and speed user, was almost five months' pregnant at the time of her interview and having a difficult time deciding what to do. She had aborted several times in the past and spoke at length about feeling tremendous guilt. Nevertheless, she was under constant pressure from her friends to have another abortion. Cheryll's friend told her, "Go get an abortion 'cause you're not going to be dragging that baby up to my house trying to get a fix."

Another key person in many women's lives was their mother. Many of the women debated whether or not to inform their mothers because they acknowledged their mothers' influential power. Interviewees discussed their mothers' religious beliefs and how they could never have an abortion if their mothers found out about the pregnancy. A much smaller group of interviewees' mothers (four) urged their daughters to abort and threatened to withdraw support if they continued their pregnancies. In this respect, the grandmothers-to-be had considerable power, particularly for those women who were living with their mothers and dependent upon their good will and generosity.

Many conflicting emotions accompanied the discovery of pregnancy. The women had to address their own joy, sorrow, surprise, ambivalence—and they had to manage the reactions of those around them.

The Private Dilemma

Once the pregnancy was acknowledged or confirmed by a pregnancy test, the question of whether or not to have an abortion moved squarely to the forefront of the women's previously private debate. The reaction of abusive partners frightened many women. As Sylvia, a thirty-six-year-old African American, said, "He told me he would kill me if I had an abortion. He says if I killed the baby, he was going to kill me."

Conversely, some men wanted the women to abort and

used violence or threats of violence to coerce them. Heather detailed her partner's reaction:

> He bitched and hollered, "I never wanted any kids. You tricked me." [Then she kicked him out.] Then all the big-time stuff started. He kicked my door in, breaking and entering my apartment. He started taking me to court trying to get custody of our son. He started getting in front of me on a back road going to work. He would drive in front of me so I couldn't pass him and make me late for work. Finally, he beat the shit out of me, maimed me. I missed the first day after the New Year of going back to work 'cause I had to go to the doctor. I got a note, went to work, gave it to my boss. He was upset that I had a note, but he said he guessed he had to let me do some light work. I was on my feet all of the time. I did chemical processing, and I had to lift heavy things of acids, which I could not do because my leg was that swollen. I lost my job.

Some women found the abortion dilemma so difficult they tried to ignore the signs of pregnancy—for example, Chloe and Thelma.

> *Chloe:* I thought, "Maybe I'll have a miscarriage." I just didn't think. I was like, "Maybe I'm just nervous. My nerves are bad and my period ain't come yet." I'm trying to find every excuse not to think that I was pregnant, and I refused to go to the doctor. So I was like, "I'm not pregnant."

> *Thelma:* I pretty much knew, but I guess I didn't want to believe it. I don't want to be. You try to make it, like make believe you're not pregnant.

In some cases, the women delayed making a decision until the stage in pregnancy in which a safe/legal abortion was no longer possible or they were so far along in the pregnancy that they did not feel they should terminate. These delays reflected the ambivalence that many women expressed regarding their pregnancies. Additionally, a number of women commented on the way time passed so quickly when they were using drugs.

> *Lindley:* Yeah, it [time] do go faster, because before you know it, a month or two have passed and you're like, "I'm still doing the same shit. Damn!"

> *Chelsea:* It goes really fast. It's like, Whew! And you really aren't doing anything. It's not like it's a constant smoking. It's just the time. You know you have to have something done, a responsibility done, and you don't get there. But you're looking at your watch and it just—whew!

For these women, the decision was made by default; abortion ceased to be an alternative. Again, the question of control is crucial. For women whose lives had been characterized by disappointments and failed plans, *not* planning was a logical response. As one woman articulated eloquently, "Things always come out differently than I expect. So I don't expect."

In addition to the women who were too far along in their pregnancies to have an abortion, some women were opposed to abortion on religious grounds. Karene, a thirty-year-old African American, was five months' pregnant with her third child. Her two oldest children had been placed in foster care, and she told the interviewer how hard that was for her. Although the father of this baby left her when she told him she was pregnant, abortion was still not an acceptable option for Karene: "I was more scared of having an abortion than I was of having [the baby], because I say, 'Well, the Lord, he'll take me. He could take me just as quick as in getting an abortion as he can me having the baby. I'm killing something, you know. I'm taking a life,' I say."

Darleen had similar concerns when she was five months' pregnant. She had already aborted two pregnancies. These were tough decisions for her because abortion was against her Islamic faith. The men she was with were abusive, however, and she could not bring a child into the world under those conditions. During her interview, Darleen explained why she decided to continue with her third pregnancy: "I'm not having an abortion because then I might not be able to have any children, and so I can see what I looked like when I was little." She also expressed concern about the effects of her crack use on the baby: "I'm praying that my child does not come out fucked up. But if he does, I'll still keep him. It'll be my child."

While Darleen reconciled herself to accepting her child regardless of any possible drug-related damage, for the other women the possibility of impairment prompted them to seek an abortion. Once the decision to terminate was made, however, further obstacles arose. Their health care options were limited due to their status as drug users as well as their lack of financial resources.

Naomi used speed and heroin for many years. After the birth of her son, she wrongly assumed she would not need birth control while she breastfed. She became pregnant shortly after the birth and knew she needed to have an abortion: "I did actually end up having an abortion after I was pregnant, which was like so traumatic for me. It was horrible. And I was discriminated against because I told the truth. They asked me about my history."

On the day her abortion was scheduled, a clinic staff member called Naomi and told her they could not perform her abortion because of her history of injection drug use. At this point, she was several months' pregnant and knew she could not wait much longer. After calling a number of hospitals and clinics, she finally lied about her drug use and found a provider to perform the abortion. She told her interviewer: "I was pretty shocked when I was discriminated against. I mean, usually when you're honest, you know, you can work something out."

Similarly, Liz, who had a daily heroin habit, had an abortion three weeks before her interview. She had difficulty locating a provider, and the entire experience proved to be extremely unpleasant:

> I wish that health care was a lot more accessible for women in this country. . . . The people in hospitals, doctors and nurses, just treat drug addicts really badly. I think that's really unfair. . . . I can't be totally honest. I can't go into a doctor's office and say, "Look, I'm a heroin addict," to tell them everything that I need to tell them about what I've done to my body and my health. I don't think there is a doctor in this city that I can go to that I can be comfortable with and they can be comfortable with me and treat me totally equal as anybody else, you know?

The decision to terminate a pregnancy was made amid a barrage of conflicting emotions, including fears of aborting or of giving birth to a drug-damaged infant. Our interviewees anguished over the potential responses to their pregnancies by the important people in their lives and suffered when their significant others did not support their decisions or tried to force them to make a decision. Many abusive partners tightened their control on the women's already constricted lives. Despite the cacophony of advice, threats, and emotions, most (112) of our interviewees continued their pregnancies.

"Like the Ember of a Fire": Opportunity, Hope, and Resolve

Pregnancy offered a chance at motherhood—possibly one of the only conventional, socially sanctioned identities available to the women in our study. From the child who endured incest, to the teenager who dropped out of school, to the adult living in a dilapidated housing project and turning tricks to buy the next fix or rock, these women lived with what Goffman (1963) called chronically spoiled identities. The role of mother, given the theoretically hallowed place it occupies in our society's cultural imagery, was a potential source of hope and pride.

For those women who had already been mothers and lost custody of their older children, the decision to have another baby was another chance at being a "good mother." Their decisions not to abort were often influenced by their guilt and remorse over past abortions or for having failed in the past. The baby-to-be became an opportunity to do it right this time.

Valerie Raskin (1992) interviewed fifteen low-income women in Chicago's inner city who were pregnant or had recently delivered and had been referred for substance abuse consultation. Raskin portrayed the double loss of losing custody of a child:

> The loss of one's children is at once both the loss of a loved person and the loss of an abstraction. One loses one's baby or child(ren) and one's ideal image of oneself as a competent mother. (1992, 149)

> A common maladaptive response seen in perinatal loss and involuntary custody loss is rapid subsequent pregnancy in an effort to replace the lost baby. (1992, 151)

Given the conflation of the images of woman and mother in American culture, to fail at motherhood is to fail at what is considered a woman's most fundamental social role. What Raskin termed the "replacement baby" phenomenon also held true for our interviewees. Women who had relinquished custody to other family members or had officially lost custody of older children often expressed determination to be a better mother for this child. They were going to keep *this* baby.

While some women felt their pregnancies were yet another complication in already tenuous life circumstances, others resolved to change their lives. Many women, such as Rhonda, felt that concern for their babies could motivate them and their partners to either cut down or quit their drug use altogether: "I tried my best to get pregnant by this guy I was with. [I] could not get pregnant for a whole year. Because I know if I get pregnant, I could stop the drug. This was the only way I could stop."

In fact, some women, such as Bridget, felt that their pregnancies were a form of divine intervention: "I found out I was pregnant. And to me it was like a message from God saying, 'Okay, now I'm giving you one more chance. If you blow this, your ass is out.'"

"Out to Here": Changes Brought about by Visible Pregnancy

If the discovery of pregnancy was accompanied by a barrage of advice from family and friends, visibly pregnant women found that the social commentary had only just begun. The stigma that members of conventional society confer on pregnant addicts is just as virulent in drug-using scenes. It became painfully clear to these women that their pregnancies bore scant resemblance to the idealized mother-to-be of modern magazines—happily knitting booties in well-appointed, sunlit rooms. Additionally, like other pregnant women, their expanding stomachs were something to be commented upon and touched by friends, acquaintances, and even strangers. Emily Martin's (1987) work on the power of the Marxist metaphor in understanding underlying cultural assumptions about the relations of reproduction helps us to understand pregnant drug users' unique social position. Continuing Martin's metaphor, pregnant drug users purposely poisoned their means of production. Our interviewees paid dearly for such violations.

Stigma

When visibly showing and publicly using drugs, the women were stigmatized in almost every social situation, including sex work and drug-use procurement settings. Stigmatization expanded their feelings of guilt and fear. When women were "out to here," they found themselves even more dependent upon their partners and vulnerable to violence.

As we have noted, many interviewees worked as prostitutes to earn enough money to survive. Sex work while pregnant, however, proved to be even more complicated and problematic. Darleen continued to prostitute while pregnant since sex work was her major source of income:

I've had sex a few times, but I don't have sex with just anybody. But me being like humungo [huge] . . . I've just had it a few times. I couldn't catch a date 'cause I was pregnant. [It's harder to catch dates] 'cause I don't dress like I used to. I don't wear any ho' clothes like I used to. I'm more casual and just wear looser clothes. But I don't do that much, 'cause if what's his name see me out there . . . he *really* don't like that, when I'm pregnant especially. He's got the whole TL [Tender-loin District] watching me.

The inability to work as much as before the pregnancy had financial implications for the women's entire house-holds. It often created a situation in which women became more dependent upon their partners, who in turn had the potential to become even more abusive. Other actors in their social scenes (associates, potential tricks, and drug dealers) called them pejorative names and generally considered their continued sex work to be scandalous.

Visible pregnancy also had implications for the women's drug use. The women we interviewed often found that drug dealers would either refuse to sell to them or berate them loudly, at length and publicly, before conducting business. Some women found this so distressing that they relied upon their partners to purchase their drugs, further increasing their dependence. Veronica explained, "Oh, people are re-ally strong against being pregnant, especially big pregnant, and they see them out there using. A lot of dope dealers will not sell to pregnant women . . . 'cause when you are stick-ing out like that, a lot of people look down on you. I, my-self, would not sell to women that are pregnant."

Many PAD participants cast aspersions on other preg-nant drug users. Veronica contended:

And especially using coke while you're pregnant . . . 'cause I know a few girls that are out there working the streets, using a lot of coke and heroin, but they don't care about even thinking about trying to clean up or thinking about getting on methadone. Those are the ones I don't have no respect for 'cause they don't even try. I mean, can you imagine going with a guy [conducting sex work] being eight, nine months' preg-nant? I can't see it. And a lot of girls do it. That's when you lose respect for them, and you just don't even want to talk to them because they don't care about themselves or that baby.

As a result of the disapproval of others who were participating in activities in which they themselves were involved, most women differentiated themselves according to their level of guilt. Darleen distinguished herself from the other crack "monsters":

> She smokes crack like this. . . . I mean, she doesn't even care. Like she's *way* out here. And then she smokes crack constantly, constantly, and she doesn't even give a, you know. I mean, I know, at least I feel guilty. I know I shouldn't be doing what I'm doing. I'm just getting tired of going down there. I'm homeless. [But] what can you do? 'cause, I mean, me on the street pregnant? Uh, uh! It's just not right.

One result of the public stigmatization of visibly pregnant drug users was women's fear of loss of custody. For example, at the time of her interview, Veronica estimated that she was about three months' pregnant with her fifth child. She was using crack, heroin, and alcohol. Her financial situation worsened when her partner's drug use escalated and he lost his job. They were living together in an SRO hotel. Child Protective Services had taken her other children, and she was fearful her pregnancy would be discovered and she would lose this baby as well:

> It's really hard 'cause once they get them [the babies], it's hard to get them back. Yeah, once they know about you, they're always gonna keep an eye on you every minute. It's like from the first time they get the phone call from the methadone people, they always watch you no matter what. They just keep close tabs on you.

Violence

More than one-third (36 percent) of the women in our study reported that they had been abused during their current (at the time of interview) pregnancy. Darleen's partner had her in the proverbial Catch 22. Her sex work was their primary source of income; however, when she came home from work, he would beat her for both dating and using drugs. In an effort to pacify him, she made an effort to bring home either money or a few crack rocks. Although this strategy sometimes worked, she could never be certain when he would become violent and begin beating her anyway. Ironically, the women explained, the combination of pregnancy and battering drastically diminished a woman's worth in the sexual marketplace. Damaged physical capital (the sex worker's body) reduced earning potential. Darleen shared her bewilderment:

> I mean, it don't make any sense either. If you got somebody . . . it's like, if a pimp's got a girl working for him, it doesn't make sense to be hitting her all in the face and then putting her out on the street. Nobody's gonna want her then. Nobody's gonna want a beat-up old broad, you know what I'm saying? It doesn't even make sense.

Although Darleen's partner was excited about her pregnancy and the baby, he also began to admonish her regarding her drug use. In addition to his verbal interventions, he threatened to hurt her if she did not stop smoking crack: "Well, I know I'm not gonna take too much hitting. You know, he hasn't hit me in like a month. When I'm pregnant it's like [he says], 'I'll hit you in your stomach.'"

All too often violence extended well beyond verbal threats into outright battering. For example, two interviewees were battered until they miscarried. Eliza was raised in south-central Los Angeles. Violence was a major part of her childhood as well as her adult relationships. She talked about the children's father and how much more difficult life was when he used drugs. Drug use made him even more violent. When Eliza became pregnant with twins, he said to her, "Don't you know I'll kill you and them babies, too?" Eventually, he beat her so badly she was hospitalized. Eliza's physician instructed her to return home and put up her feet because she would most likely miscarry.

> My body started just hurting real bad. I started bleeding, and I just couldn't move. So I called my sister, and I asked her if she would take me to the hospital, and she did. And the next thing I remember is waking up in the bed and the hospital priest was praying over me. That's when it hit me that this man don't care for me. He told me he'd kill me and these babies, too. Well, the babies was dead. They was gone and dead and gone. I mean, he put his knee all the way into my stomach. Hey, there's no way they could have survived. And I thought about what he had said, and I remember seeing the priest walk out. And I thought, he meant what he said. That's when I learned to take a man at his word when he tells you something. I wanted to go out and get a gun and kill him. But some people can kill and some people can't.

When we interviewed her, Doris was seven months' pregnant. She was living alone in a Catholic sanctuary and planned to enroll in a drug treatment program to "get her life together" and regain custody of her children. She talked about the father of her two youngest children:

> He abused me for three years. He had me out there on the ho' stro' [whore stroll] making money for his habit.

He's broken my jaw. He broke it twice within a week. He came across my back with a hammer. I was pregnant with twins, but my daughter twin didn't make it. I actually pushed out a deceased body because when he hit me across my back with that hammer, he fractured the baby's skull. So I carried around a dead fetus for two and a half months. No matter how many charges I pressed, they was never pressed. Everything was thrown out. You know how they say they're gonna beat the shit out of you? I actually had the shit beat out of me. And the police officer could smell it on me.

Many kinds of abuse contributed to the troubled trajectory of pregnancy, not only drug abuse but physical, emotional, and sexual abuse as well. The majority of pregnancies were unplanned, and the discovery process was characterized by mixed emotions—guilt, fear, and ambivalence as well as hope. In the later stages of pregnancy, when women were showing, many changes took place in their lives. The women then publicly occupied two incompatible statuses: mother-to-be and drug user.

4

Harm

Perception

and Harm

Reduction

Once they learned they were pregnant, all of the women in our study began to worry that their drug use had already damaged their developing fetuses. Some women had witnessed, or had heard about, other pregnant drug users who had given birth to less than healthy babies. We learned, however, that women relied to a lesser extent on their personal knowledge and experience. Like most Americans, our study participants' views were shaped largely by media accounts of drugs' harmful effects on the fetus. Given the time period of our data collection, 1991–94, it is not surprising that crack users were most convinced of the inevitability of their babies suffering from drug-related harm.

Only eight interviewees (7 percent) responded to pregnancy by having an abortion.[1] The rest continued their pregnancies and continued to use drugs. Most women, however, changed their behavior in ways they hoped would reduce further harm. Typically, women decreased drug consumption or switched to drugs they believed were less dangerous. Women tried to improve their health by eating better, sleeping more, or taking prenatal vitamins. Some women sought prenatal care, others drug treatment. All of the women, at times, held fatalistic attitudes about their babies' well-being; but to varying degrees, most also made attempts to put their babies' health ahead of their own immediate needs and desires.

Sasha, a twenty-four-year-old African-American crack smoker in her seventh month of pregnancy, had resigned herself to her continued addictive drug use. Nonetheless, she was aware of her capacity to make better rather than worse choices: "I know I'm an addict, and I do like to get high, but I don't want to die, you know what I'm saying? So in my mind—this is my own philosophy—if you're gonna do it, you need to know when you're getting close to the edge and try to back up a little bit."

Amanda, who was six months' pregnant, had adopted a similar philosophy. Although she continued to smoke crack intermittently, her pregnancy led her to pay attention to the hazards of her drug-involved life-style:

> Okay, I got a problem with drugs. Okay, fine. I gotta do something. But in the moment when I'm doing this drug, I am aware of my life. I'm not just focusing on this drug. I'm not just focusing on this hit, because when your mind becomes so involved with that hit, you forget about somebody coming up on you killing you. You forget about all these things until something drastic happens like, I'm six feet under, or God, my baby's dead. I'm going to jail, or I just got stabbed. That's very, very dangerous. There's a way to do this. There's

a way. If you're gonna do it, do it in the right manner as to where you're caring for your life.

For Amanda, harm reduction involved little more than thinking about "all these things." Nonetheless, her growing awareness of the dangers of drugs to herself and her baby represented an important change in her thinking about her drug choices. Unfortunately, Amanda, like Sasha, believed there was nothing she could do to lower substantially the risk of having a crack-damaged baby. As the rest of the chapter illustrates, women's belief in the inevitability and irreversibility of fetal harm often served as an obstacle to their adopting more comprehensive harm-reduction practices.

Harm Perception

Interviewees' degree of concern about newborn outcomes varied according to their primary drug of choice. Crack users were the most frightened. At the time these interviews were conducted, the media buzz surrounding crack use was tremendous (Humphries 1999, Reinarman and Levine 1989). Subsequent research shows that early media reports grossly exaggerated crack's dangers (Barth 1991, Chasnoff et al. 1992, Coles et al. 1992, Lutiger et al. 1991). Drugs such as marijuana, heroin, and methamphetamine received much less media attention; as a result, women who used these drugs were uncertain about potential harm to their babies.

Sociologist Troy Duster (1970) described the ways in which moral panics about particular drugs relate to public perceptions regarding the race and class of the people who use them. Clearly, the social construction of crack as a demon drug was predicated on images of the typical crack user as a low-income, African-American urban dweller (Humphries

1999, Reinarman and Levine 1997).[2] Feminist scholars also remind us that central to this same panic was the social and medical construction of the mother's body as toxic to her fetus (Chavkin 1991, Fink 1990, Harrison 1991, Muraskin 1991). Thus, the ease with which Americans—including the women in this study—came to accept the worst-case scenario of crack's detrimental effect on the fetus must be understood within the context of institutional sexism and racism. Interviewees who used heroin or methamphetamine worried about the effects of their drug use on their babies-to-be; however, women who used crack, 82 percent of whom were African American, clearly expressed the gravest concerns.

Crack

Typical of the crack users in our study, Sasha and Amanda used crack in binges. Crack binges were characterized by the women smoking one crack rock after another in a process called "smoking back to back." Such smoking could last for several days, during which the women ate and slept minimally if at all. Participants referred to this use pattern as "going on 24/7," which meant smoking twenty-four hours a day, seven days a week. While 24/7 was a common expression, the women almost never actually went without sleep for an entire week. Most crack binges lasted no longer than three or four days. The women often interspersed periods of abstinence between binges, and such periods ranged from a few hours to a few months.

Waldorf, Reinarman, and Murphy, who studied primarily middle-class cocaine freebasers and crack smokers, conceptualized crack-using binges as episodic compulsion. Unlike addictive use patterns, episodic compulsion involves continual consumption within a single smoking episode. During an episode women would smoke back to back for hours and hours, with periods of days, weeks, and some-times months without using crack. Reinarman and col-leagues discussed differences between addictive use patterns of alcohol and heroin and the repeated bingeing of crack smokers: "What is called crack addiction then—repeatedly returning to bingeing—is comprised of volition as well as compulsion and is more a psychological matter than a phar-macological or physiological one" (1997, 79).

Episodic compulsion was a source of confusion and shame for PAD participants. There were days or weeks when they successfully left the crack pipe alone. Then the baby's father came home with a rock for them to share, or their welfare checks arrived. They were then "on a mission"—ready to start another crack-using binge. In general, crack users could not make sense of their ability to stop for a while and their inability to stop using once they had started again.

Crack's mysterious hold on them, combined with fears of fetal damage, were consistent themes in the women's narratives. Some women worried that crack use would cause their children to have serious behavioral problems, while others worried their infants would be born with deformed arms, legs, or facial features. Women also worried about the possibility of mental impairment. While the women's fears and concerns varied, crack smokers all believed that crack was certain to cause some kind of problem. Amanda, for example, felt that crack-related difficulties were unavoid-able and began early in her pregnancy to brace herself for such an outcome.

> This baby has been exposed to crack cocaine from the first beginning of conception to . . . about now, and that's what? Six months? I don't like that. That's a bad feeling, because this baby's suffered a lot of damage. Yeah, I'm mentally tripping because it's already bad

enough my son's gonna suffer in his childhood. But there's no sense in me sitting here living in a fantasy world thinking that, "Well, Amanda, you done smoke from one to six months, that amount of drugs from one to six months is not gonna have any effect on my baby even if I do quit right now." That's a lie—I know there's gonna be effects already.

Rhonda smoked one hundred dollars' worth of crack every day during the first several weeks of her pregnancy. At two months, when she saw a physician and discovered her pregnancy, she looked back with horror at the number of rocks she had smoked. She immediately quit using, but the fear of possible physiological problems haunted her. In her third month of pregnancy, Rhonda had an abortion. She took full responsibility for her decision:

> The baby was doomed from the start. I don't care what those doctors say when they say, "Oh, you're pregnant and you can stop using drugs and your body will be okay." That's a lie. 'Cause my baby suffered after that, and it was my fault, my own fault. I ain't blaming it on nothing. I'm not saying because the doctors didn't notice it or nothing. It was me.

Rhonda, like most interviewees, believed that her crack use during the first weeks of pregnancy did serious and, more important, irreversible damage. In chapter 7 we address the demise of the "crack baby" sensation and show how even babies born to mothers who smoked 24/7 were able, with proper nutrition and care, to catch up with their birth cohort. At the time of these interviews, however, both the crack smokers and the people observing them (family members, friends, social workers, doctors, researchers, journalists, and other drug users) firmly believed that crack-exposed infants could not escape serious physical and mental problems.

Heroin

The women who used heroin approached pregnancy with far less trepidation and anxiety. Heroin did not receive the same sort of media attention in the late 1980s and early 1990s, and many heroin users were confident they could deliver healthy infants. Moreover, heroin had been on the street longer than crack, and its effects were better known to drug users. Many women either had already delivered healthy heroin-exposed babies or knew other women who had done so.

Chandra was representative of this group. She was a heroin user in her fourth month of pregnancy who firmly believed that heroin caused few, if any, problems: "The heroin does not hurt them at all. All my three babies had it. As long as you eat and you sleep. See, that's the reason we wanted to participate [in the study] is just to show people that it's not the drug, it's the situation."

Later in the interview, Chandra tried to illustrate the relative harmlessness of heroin during pregnancy as compared to other drugs. Crack, she felt, was the worst drug to use while pregnant. As she said this, she grabbed a piece of paper and began drawing a picture of the typical heroin baby and a typical crack baby. The crack baby's sketch was thinner than the sketch of the heroin baby. Chandra drew dark circles under the crack-exposed infant's eyes to emphasize its compromised health.

Lauren, a nineteen-year-old white heroin user, had similar beliefs and experiences. She had used heroin during both of her previous pregnancies. When we interviewed her, Lauren was convinced that heroin did not jeopardize her chances for a healthy outcome. She espoused a "mellow drug" philosophy regarding opiate use while pregnant:

> I knew the heroin would relax the baby. And I would do codeine. I'd do Percodans [a prescription pain reliever classified as an opiate]. Those are all narcotics, class-two or -three narcotics. And these are things that just mellow you out. It goes through the bloodline and stuff, but it doesn't really cause a birth defect. But when you do crack or you do LSD or something, then you start to worry.

The women in this group had used heroin for a number of years, often during past pregnancies. Since they felt that heroin use was not a health risk, they tended to focus more on controlling their use rather than quitting entirely. In contrast to undergoing the binges and abstentions described by the crack users, most women in this group chose to maintain their drug use at lower levels during pregnancy rather than go cold turkey or attempt abrupt abstinence.

Methamphetamine

Except for one Asian woman, all the methamphetamine users were white. Speed users were most likely to express uncertainty regarding the potential impact of their drug use on themselves and their forming fetuses. Most of these women were pregnant for the first time and therefore had no prior experience to rely upon.

In the early 1990s, methamphetamine use was largely overlooked in the pregnancy and drug-use discourse. Very few studies addressed the potential problems associated with methamphetamines; even fewer media stories focused on its use during pregnancy. Perhaps as a result, women's views on methamphetamine wavered. Although none of the women could cite specific problems that might result from speed use during pregnancy, most imagined that some kind of trouble must ensue. Methamphetamine users did not eat regularly and often went without sleep for days at a time. Every woman we interviewed knew that eating and sleeping were very important for fetal health. While the crack users had quivering incubator babies to envision, and the heroin addicts could imagine a baby in classic withdrawal, the methamphetamine users lacked such specific information or images. For some women, not knowing left them to imagine the worst. For others, the lack of available information allowed them to relegate their concerns to the back of their minds.

Emily and Pamela exemplify methamphetamine users' range of responses. Emily suspected she was pregnant during her first trimester. She had used methamphetamine intermittently for the previous twelve years, first recreationally and then as a diet aid. She injected small amounts of methamphetamine three times a week. While she wished that she had more money for things other than drugs, she had no plans to quit using in the near future. Emily could not even imagine the type or severity of harm that methamphetamine use during pregnancy might cause. At one point during her interview, she asked, "I would really like to find out more about why, . . . but [I would like] any articles or stuff to read on the effects of the drug on the baby, you know, from the mother's use of drugs. I look reasonably healthy. I feel reasonably healthy."

Emily did not know where to begin to look for the information she needed. While she felt healthy, her drug use made her question whether she was hurting either herself or her fetus. Consequently, she turned to her friends, other long-term methamphetamine users, for health information: "I mean, I definitely felt guilty about it [using methamphetamines during pregnancy]. Even though he [her partner] and other people kept trying to convince me that speed isn't really harmful. Other drugs are more harmful, like alcohol or LSD or something like that. I just can't think it is going to be harmless." Like the other speed users, Emily found it difficult to articulate a specific set of possible consequences. Instead, she voiced a more general concern about potential negative effects.

Pamela had a long history of speed use and also did not plan to quit using any time in the near future. She was keenly aware of the possible problems of this type of drug use and believed that the lack of information was evidence of the dangerousness of the substance. She believed that methamphetamine users should not have children until more was known about the drug's effects on the mother and the child's health:

> These people who are doing it now . . . it's really scary. Like I said, I know what happened to the children that were subject to their parents' drinking or their mother's drinking while they were pregnant with them. Just that alone scares me. Nobody knows really what the amphetamine . . . or, see . . . that's another thing why I'm so against it being so illegal, because when it's legal they'll study it more and it'll be more open and people will find out really. People are going to use it anyway, whether they say it's okay or not. But when the alcohol studies started coming out, I know a lot of people who stopped drinking. A lot of people cut back on their drinking when they actually could see what damages . . . if you can't see what the damage is, it doesn't register. People should be able to see it. And if it's not open or it's not allowed—nobody knows what happens due to amphetamine use and pregnancy. And I've been doing those things for twenty years!

Speed's probable harms bothered Pamela's conscience. Her pregnancy was an accident, and she had made definite plans to terminate it. Since Pamela was unwilling to gamble on the uncertain nature of methamphetamine-related fetal morbidity, abortion was her only option.

Harm-Reduction Strategies

While women's particular worries varied depending on their drug of choice, one common theme emerged: all of the study participants approached pregnancy with some apprehension. While cessation of drug use was widely accepted as an ultimate goal, complete abstinence was difficult to achieve and even harder to maintain. Interviewees drew upon a repertoire of techniques to manage their fears and minimize the potential effects of their drug use.

Switching Drugs

One method that women used to diminish drug-related harm was to use lesser amounts of their drug of choice, often combining or substituting another drug that they believed to be less harmful. This harm-reduction strategy was most frequently implemented by the crack users, reflecting their heightened concerns regarding the impact of crack on their babies.

Sasha substituted marijuana for crack while pregnant. She described her strategy: "Yeah, I couldn't do anything. I just smoked pot a little bit. You know, I smoked pot. He [her husband] knew I did have a drug problem, okay, so what he would do if he seen me getting edgy or what, he'd say, 'Go in my closet, dear. I got some weed in there. Why don't you smoke some of that.'"

Darleen's crack smoking was "putting worry" on her. She feared her child might be born with "a hole in its heart or something." She mixed crack with marijuana to decrease her crack intake: "Well, so now I've got to smoking more weed than crack. And then if I do get some crack, I'm gonna get like three rocks and maybe just roll up three rocks. And if I roll me some weed, it's gonna keep me high all day long." Darleen's strategy successfully interrupted her compulsive back-to-back crack-smoking pattern while it increased her marijuana use.

In addition to drug switching, some women tried to have on and off days. Denise, a twenty-three-year-old crack smoker, explained this method: "I mean, with the baby I shouldn't be getting high anyway. We all know that's a no-no. I be . . . okay, that's two weeks I haven't smoked, so that's two weeks for the baby. Now I can get high. Then I'll have two more weeks. You gotta think like that."

Counteracting Drug Use

Since women's attempts to reduce or stop their drug use were not always successful, they employed other methods to try to reduce harm. These were strategies for counteracting drug use. PAD participants consumed substances they believed could cleanse their systems of drug-related toxins. They ingested prenatal vitamins, niacin, pickle juice, and vinegar for this purpose. Peggy, for example, was a crack smoker who wanted to be clean when she had her third child. The night before her interview she threw away all her crack pipes and began drinking pickle juice: "I been drinking a lot of pickle juice and eating a lot of pickles. 'Cause that cleans your system out. Yeah, I been drinking vinegar, too. I been drinking vinegar straight now with a little warm water. I'm gonna make sure there ain't nothing in my system with this one."

Women also believed that vinegar, goldenseal, and pickle juice would speed up the body processes for eliminating evidence of their drug use. They employed these methods to facilitate providing a drug-free urinalysis to their health care provider. In chapter 5 we discuss how from some women's perspectives hiding drug use from health and social welfare agents was a form of harm reduction.

Many women believed that prenatal vitamins were very important for their babies' development. Even the women who did not attend prenatal care purchased prenatal vitamins and proudly reported to us how faithfully they took them. In some women's narratives, prenatal vitamins seemed to almost play the role of magic bullets. Women imbued them with the power to undo their negative health behaviors. A recurring theme in these interviews was that continued drug use was indeed scandalous. But taking vitamins was something the women were doing for the baby. Even if they continued to use what they (and almost everyone else in their lives) believed were very injurious drugs, they hoped (and often prayed) that the vitamins would help their babies to be healthy.

Altering Drug-using Life-styles

Women knew that their life-styles were not good for their babies-to-be. Acquiring money for drugs, buying drugs, taking drugs, and coming down from drug highs all compromised their health. Although the women acknowledged and put up with these potentially dangerous activities when they were not pregnant, pregnancy was a time when they tried to change as many unhealthy routines as possible. They were particularly conscious of any health hazards that could compound the already deleterious qualities of their drug consumption.

Whether pharmacologically induced or the result of drug expenses, poor eating habits accompanied inundation into drug-using life-styles. Women understood that poor nutrition was a serious problem for growing babies-to-be. On a regular basis, most women forced themselves to eat the best food they could find. For example, when Amanda smoked crack, she constantly struggled with her lack of appetite. She explained her views on eating regularly as a harm-reduction strategy:

> I had to eat. I had to put something in my baby's system so the drug won't affect him or hit him as hard, because I can't see that. I cannot see knowing you have a weakness and sitting up there smoking and knowing you have a life in you, too, at the same time and not feeding your child, because what that boil down to is . . . yeah, I know I'm hurting my child. But if you know that your weakness is there, you're going to try to help your child at the same time. You're gonna feed it. Even though you're doing something wrong, even though you're doing something that is not basically right and you have no control over the drug or the weaknesses that you have, you have control whether you feed your child while he's inside you.

PAD Project participants were also well aware of the importance of getting enough sleep. To be able to sleep regularly, women needed to move away from friends or family members who were using drugs or leave drug-saturated neighborhoods. Sasha tried numerous times to reduce her crack use but continually failed because her husband and most of the other people living in her building were avid crack smokers. She lived in one of San Francisco's biggest public housing projects, which was well known for its open drug use and sales. Before her pregnancy, her apartment was a "crack house"—a place where people came to smoke in private or sell crack. They often "kicked her down," giving her a rock or two as payment for using her apartment. After

Sasha discovered her pregnancy, she realized that this routine would ruin her chances of having a healthy baby. She outlined her attempts to juggle life in "a little rock house" with concerns for her baby-to-be:

> *Sasha:* I was approximately four months' pregnant. And that's when it just, just being around it, easy access to it, not having to pay for it every day. People would, "Hey, can I come in here and smoke?"
>
> *Interviewer:* And they'll pay you?
>
> *Sasha:* Drugs or money. It was like on every floor, and there's twenty floors. It's just easy access, and it was constantly every day [knocks on a table to imitate a person knocking on a door] somebody's knocking at my door. And from morning to night, I just had a little rock house. You know what I'm saying? But I didn't sell drugs.
>
> *Interviewer:* So what were your eating and sleeping habits like at that time?
>
> *Sasha:* Very poor. Very poor. I knew what I had to do was I had to eat before somebody knocked on the door. So when I would get up in the morning, I'd rush to the kitchen and try to get stuff in me, food in me, take my prenatal vitamins and that's about it. I just would take my vitamins and eat a little bit.

Our interviewees shared the same problems faced by other poor pregnant women who need decent nutritious food and safe, relatively stable, and quiet housing. Their situations were exacerbated by the resources they depleted buying costly drugs and the loss of appetite and wakefulness brought on by drug intoxication. When they could, they moved out of living situations inundated with drug users and sellers. Almost all of the interviewees, however, were forced by their financial situations to try to implement available harm-reduction strategies among people and in places that challenged the most committed mother-to-be.

Prenatal Care

Findings from general population studies of pregnant women indicate that reasons for lack of prenatal care attendance include financial barriers (Gold, Kenney, and Singh 1987); blocks to access due to distance, lack of child care, language barriers, or unfamiliarity with health care systems (Miller, Downs, and Testa 1989); perceived unimportance of care when pregnancy seems normal (Fisher et al. 1991; Patterson, Freese, and Goldenberg 1990); denial, depression, ambivalence, or unhappiness about the pregnancy (Fisher et al. 1991, Pettiti and Coleman 1990); and lack of awareness of pregnancy in early months (Burks 1992, Sable et al. 1990).[3] In addition, pregnant drug users have unique barriers to health care that have received little research attention. In a previous study of heroin users, we found that lack of awareness of pregnancy due to drug-related amenorrhea (irregular menses) caused delays in seeking prenatal care. Further, stigmatization of pregnant drug users by health care workers made them reluctant to access care (Rosenbaum 1979). Fear of imprisonment or loss of child custody has been suggested as a barrier to care for pregnant cocaine users (Chavkin and Kandall 1990; York, Williams, and Munro 1993), but to date little empirical evidence has been available to support this claim.

The association between drug use and lack of prenatal care has become so widely accepted that urban hospitals routinely conduct drug tests on pregnant women admitted with incomplete prenatal care attendance (Land and Kushner 1990, McCalla et al. 1991). Nonetheless, all of our interviewees believed that prenatal care was one of the most important means to improved fetal health. With very few exceptions, the women who believed that their drug use posed grave threats to fetal well-being also had very problematic relationships with prenatal care providers. For women who sought prenatal care, the question of whether or not to disclose their drug use had to be addressed. While the medical literature indicates that lack of prenatal care may put a woman at risk for a poor pregnancy outcome, from the drug-using woman's perspective, seeking prenatal care might also put her at risk of losing her child if her drug habit were detected. In short, the dilemma is as follows: not to disclose may compromise the baby's health, but disclosure may result in loss of custody. Weighing these risks was a major challenge for women. The crack users, most fearful of fetal damage, focused on the importance of prenatal care as a health concern. Heroin users, on the other hand, were less concerned about fetal damage and more fearful of loss of custody. Methamphetamine users, having no information at all, were characterized by uncertainty.

More than half of the sample participated to some degree in prenatal care. Pregnant drug users' decisions to attend or avoid care, both in general and on any given day, were based on their evaluation of the best way of evading threats of harm to themselves as mothers and to their infants. Both concrete problems (such as physical damage to the fetus or loss of custody) and emotional difficulties (such as stigmatization) were considered in this process.

Health Concerns. Overall, women disclosed their drug use to health care providers to enlist their cooperation in maximizing healthy pregnancies. They saw providers' medical expertise and obstetrical technology as powerful harm-reduction resources.

In her seventh month of pregnancy, Maria recalled the following conversation with her doctor: "I told my doctor, I said, 'Please have all your important instruments near you, because I used [crack] with my baby.'"

Amanda disclosed her crack use as a way of alerting her

doctor to her high-risk pregnancy. In addition to relying on technological advances, she felt that her providers could give her valuable information. She characterized her doctor-patient relationship: "When I go to my prenatal care appointment, I'll tell the doctor, 'I fucked up. I smoked. Is my baby okay?' I don't want nothing to happen to my baby. I'm learning and wanting to know all these things so it'll help me further help my baby."

For Amanda and the other women who disclosed, telling providers about their drug use during pregnancy was viewed as a way to open doors to important resources. While the women knew that prenatal caregivers could not erase crack-related harms, they believed that prenatal care was an essential step in monitoring and managing risk.

Unfortunately, the women's attempts to improve their health through traditional health care were problematic. Crack users often found that after disclosing their drug-using status they suffered harsh judgments from health care professionals. When we interviewed her, Jessie had just given birth to her first crack-exposed child. The uncomfortable memories of her hospital experiences were still fresh in her mind. During Jessie's first two pregnancies, she had not smoked crack, nor had she missed a single prenatal appointment. At delivery, her doctors and nurses were very supportive. Jessie's crack-involved pregnancy was a markedly different experience. She had smoked crack almost continuously and only managed to attend two prenatal care appointments. During labor and delivery, the doctors and nurses treated her like "a dirty little crack addict." Looking back at her own experiences and those of others, Jessie explained to her interviewer why women in her position fail to get prenatal care:

> I know a lot of mothers say that they don't get prena-
> tal care 'cause they feel like as soon as they walk

through the door they will be judged. "Oh, you're a crackhead. Why the hell did you get pregnant anyway?" So they don't get prenatal care. They have those commercials about addicts that don't get prenatal care because they just don't give a shit. They do give a shit, but they are thinking about how they gonna be looked at when they walk in the hospital door, like they were not good enough to be pregnant.

Jackie had a three-year-old and a four-month-old, both sons. She had numerous miscarriages before giving birth to her children. Jackie had been honest with the doctors about her drug use, but she finally stopped keeping her prenatal care appointments because they kept giving her "funny looks." She had disclosed her drug use because "it was like no secret. I wasn't trying to hide it, 'cause soon as they took my urine they was gonna know anyway. Every time you go for your pregnancy, they take it, yeah, and they test it for drugs."

When a woman weighed the costs and benefits of seeking prenatal care, many factors informed her decision. The value of prenatal care was considered in terms of the risks of attendance and disclosure of drug use. As the following excerpts illustrate, the women had varied experiences with health care providers; some were positive, and others were devastating.

Oprah remembered:

I'd go in one door and come out the other door, and I'd say I went to the doctor. I just didn't like them sitting up there all the time asking these same questions, and they don't check you. They just listen to the baby's heart and all that. I can listen to his heart 'cause he's inside me. I feel him. That was always good in case something was wrong. They wanted me to take a sonogram, but I didn't never go. I thought I had better things to do.

Moira held similar views: "I don't think they help you out at all. It's like they push you on the stomach. They do a urine test every time you go in. 'All right, you're doing fine. See you next month.' So I don't think I get no help from them at all."

As we noted previously, women frequently did not realize they were pregnant until they were well into their second trimester. Many women worried that coming to prenatal care when they were so far along would be held against them. Courtney's story exemplifies this "too far along" problem. When we interviewed Courtney, she was nineteen weeks' pregnant with her first child. She smoked crack and drank beer. This pregnancy was not planned, but she was very excited about having a baby. The baby started moving a week before the interview, which she told us increased her resolve to stop using drugs. But whether or not to initiate prenatal care presented Courtney with a real dilemma: "Now, if I waited till I was five months' pregnant to start prenatal, they'll test [my urine] then. It's like [prenatal care providers will think], 'Why didn't she come in? She should have come in.'"

Lavinia gave birth to her third son four months before her interview. A working-class San Franciscan, Lavinia did not start using heroin until she was twenty-seven years old. She felt that her drug use was prompted by her rape, which left her devastated for more than a year. In fact, for eight months after the rape, she was unable to leave the house. While she abstained from drugs during the last three months of her pregnancy, Lavinia had used heroin and crack during her first two trimesters. She shared her health care provider experiences: "Like, when I was in San Diego, it was hard even for me to find a doctor, because all they told me to do was get an abortion. They wouldn't deal with me." Despite this punitive treatment Lavinia was determined to receive prenatal care: "I knew that if I wasn't getting prenatal care, that would be a strike against me, since I was getting it so late."

The women who were stigmatized soon after their pregnancies were diagnosed were reluctant to continue prenatal care attendance and endure further humiliation. They were forced to navigate a precarious path between their efforts to reduce drug-related harms and to avoid stigmatization. While very few women avoided obstetric care (pre- and postnatal care) altogether, many admitted that they did not receive as much care as they would have liked.

In contrast, consider Jocylene, a twenty-six-year-old African American who was HIV positive. While she had certainly experienced discriminatory health care in the past, during her pregnancy the nurse practitioner was extremely supportive. In a powerful endorsement for understanding health care providers, Jocylene praised her doctor: "I know she is worried about me. If it wasn't for her, I'd be dead right now. People just don't understand. . . . Just a little bit of kindness can do a fucking lot. It really can."

In light of past negative health care experiences, difficulties with transportation or child care, hours spent trying to obtain public assistance and then to locate a provider who would accept the woman as a patient, it was not surprising that prenatal care received mixed reviews from our study population. As Jocylene's narrative makes clear, however, one tolerant health professional can heal more than just an ailing body. In fact, the most powerful harm-reduction strategy may be tolerant and compassionate care by practitioners with an understanding of drug users and their related life-style issues and the leeway to provide information and interventions appropriate to each patient's needs.

Custody Concerns. Heroin users, like crack users, took vitamins, went to prenatal appointments, and tried to maintain regular eating and sleeping patterns. They engaged in these activities as a way to *improve* their health during pregnancy, as opposed to the crack-using women, who hoped these health routines would *counteract* negative drug effects.

Prenatal care as a health-maintaining regimen was problematic for heroin-using women since they did not consider providers to be necessary helping agents in the process of producing a healthy baby. These women were more likely to view health care providers as extensions of Child Protective Services (CPS) who could challenge women's continued custody of the baby-to-be as well as their older children.

Among pregnant heroin users, potential loss of custody was the paramount concern. For these women *harm* was defined as loss of custody, so their harm-reduction efforts focused on reducing institutional intervention into their lives. Harm-reduction strategies included lying to providers about drug use, covering up signs of drug use, and avoiding health care all together.

Mindy, a tall, slender woman, gave birth a few days before her interview. She avoided health care until delivery because she feared health care providers would discover her drug use. Mindy managed to conceal her drug-using identity while she was in the hospital: "With L., the middle baby, the little boy, when I went to the hospital, I got my arm up in a bandage. [I said] that I had sprung my elbow or something. I made up something. I told them I just came out here from Arkansas and I had all my prenatal up there."

By "getting [her] arm up in a bandage," Mindy avoided exposing her injection scars to the hospital staff. Since she was aware that the standard profile used to identify a pregnant drug user by labor and delivery staff included lack of prenatal care, she made up a story about out-of-state prenatal care attendance. This story provided her with a reasonable alibi for presenting in labor with no medical records and allayed the staff's suspicions.

Unlike Mindy, Tanya did not feel comfortable avoiding prenatal care. Like many women in this group, however, she desperately hoped to hide her drug use from her nurses and physicians. Instead of covering up injection marks, she chose to inject in less noticeable body areas: "Mostly now I muscle [inject subcutaneously]. I just muscle it in my ass. But I mean, I've had enough to where if my doctors are gonna check me, they're not gonna tell me, 'Okay, let me see your rear.' I've even done it into my tongue."

Tanya chose to avoid intentionally or unintentionally disclosing her drug use to providers. On the other hand, she did not like lying to her doctor. Her preference was to evade being asked about her drug use. She was convinced that injecting in her buttocks and under her tongue disguised her injection drug user status from her caregivers.

Sidney and Chandra chose a radically different path from the other interviewees. Both chose to avoid prenatal care and planned to give birth outside of the hospital. Chandra had spent some time researching home births and felt confident that she and her friends could manage the birth on their own. She related her plans:

> I'm gonna have it at home, and then I'm gonna register the birth at about three of four months. I'm not going to—I didn't report this baby to welfare. I'm going to wait until it's born, and then they're gonna ask for a birth certificate, and at that point I'm gonna say— cause they're not tied with CPS in that sense. They're telling me what to do, and that's the point where I go to a lawyer and I say, "I had a home birth. I need a birth certificate."

Sidney, a heroin user, also planned to give birth outside of a hospital. Unlike Chandra, this choice was not based on her knowledge or confidence in home births. Rather, it was based on Sidney's past negative experiences with traditional health and human services agencies: "I don't know. I might just go out in the woods and have it. Go to Mexico and have it. Maybe I can kick. I don't know. I mean, I just don't know anymore."

In addition to not trusting nurses and physicians, Sidney was also petrified of a custody case. A few years before her interview, she was arrested for drug possession. The baby's father had recently died, and Sidney's parents refused to take custody of her two children. CPS intervened and placed her children in foster care. At the time of our interview, Sidney was still trying to regain custody of her children. Her chances appeared to be slim because of her difficulties in finding a job and locating permanent housing and her continued heroin use. In light of her past experiences, Sidney's plans to give birth in Mexico or in the woods seemed serious.

Uncertainty. Methamphetamine-using women were unsure of the possible problems associated with their drug use; therefore, they were less decisive than cocaine and heroin users were about which methods of harm reduction to employ. Most of these women did not know whether or not they should terminate their pregnancies. They also felt positively about health care and reported they would attend prenatal care appointments if they could make a decision about continuation or termination or if time permitted.

Pamela did not change her drug-using routine at all during pregnancy. She had made a firm decision to abort because this was the only effective harm reduction she could imagine. One month after the interview with Pamela, a PAD staff member ran into her on the street. The two talked briefly, and Pamela revealed that her plans had unexpectedly changed. The following is an excerpt from the interviewer's field notes:

> When I spoke with Pamela last month, she planned on having an abortion. At that time she felt babies should be wanted and they should have responsible healthy parents who can afford to give them whatever they want. This month her feelings on parenting and pregnancy while using speed are being tested. Being a very thin woman, I trusted her calculations that she was in the first few months of pregnancy. Unfortunately, we were both wrong. After her initial appointment for an abortion, Pamela learned she was too far along in her pregnancy to abort legally.
>
> "It just goes to show you that you never know anything about the future," was the only rationalization she could make after explaining how completely distraught this news made her. Pamela was very vague when I tried to probe into her future plans during the interview. Having an abortion was the only definite decision she could make. About other plans, she told me, " . . . things always come out differently than I expect." She's attending regular prenatal appointments now but has not quit using speed.

Sally has seven children, the youngest a two-month-old baby. She confirmed her pregnancy with an over-the-counter pregnancy test and, like Pamela, assumed she was in the first few months of pregnancy. In preparation for the baby, she and her boyfriend moved to a larger room in their residence hotel, painted the new room, moved their belongings out of storage, and collected new baby clothes. In the midst of this move, Sally began the application process for public assistance so she could begin her prenatal appointments. Unfortunately, all her work and plans were interrupted when she went into premature labor before she could attend her first appointment. Sally, too, was much further along in her pregnancy than she suspected. She described her daughter's health, premature labor, and her experiences in the hospital:

> Yeah, the lungs weren't fully developed, and they had to put her on oxygen and everything. . . . She was lethargic, which is real groggy and everything, and they said she wasn't sucking properly. You know, she wouldn't eat right. Well, I had that problem with [names second-oldest child], and it didn't have anything to do with his birth or anything else. It was they were trying to give him a bottle and he didn't want the bottle. He was a breast baby and that's all there was to it. He did not want the bottle. And we tried to talk to them at the hospital and see if maybe that was what it was with [names this baby], but they wouldn't, they didn't even want to try and find out. . . . everything was on account of the drugs. And it's like the first child care worker, Social Services, she says something about, "Well, the baby's underweight, and the baby doesn't eat well." And I said, "Well, couldn't that be due to the prematurity?" [The social worker replied,] "Yeah, or the use of drugs." And it was like they said, "Well, she's lethargic," and this, that, and the other thing, and I said, "Which could be due to her not being fully developed," and she turned around [sarcastic tone], "Well, or the use of drugs." It's like they can't actually say it's the use of drugs.

During Sally's previous pregnancies, prenatal care was a positive part of her birth experiences. Like Pamela, she had made plans, but things did not come out the way she had expected.

Pregnant crack users' participation in prenatal care was influenced by the degree to which these actions appeared to them to be useful in harm reduction. Prenatal care was an important source of support for a few, but for most it was a frightening gauntlet to be run, depending on each woman's past experiences, social network, drug-use status, and recent interactions with health care systems.

The women most in need of services—those most heavily involved in the drug life—were most alienated from prenatal care. Few felt they could disclose their drug use without risking custody loss or stigma; and many believed they would be discovered through drug testing, whether or not they disclosed. Therefore, in a context of stigmatization and fear of custody loss, the major motivation for crack users' health care participation was their own readiness to make life-style and behavioral changes, a factor over which health care practitioners had very little influence or very much help to offer.

Drug Treatment

When we interviewed them, our interviewees were not enrolled in residential or methadone drug-treatment programs. Nonetheless, many had, at some point in time, tried various drug-treatment modalities. Women believed that drug treatment only worked if the woman was ready to stop using drugs and she chose to enter a program. Nevertheless, even for those women who were receptive to the idea of drug treatment, the availability of a quality program was hardly guaranteed. Aside from a handful of tiny residential programs (usually six to ten beds), there was a paucity of available treatment for crack users. Methadone maintenance, of course, remained the prevalent option for heroin users. In the early 1990s in California, the availability of methadone treatment slots, even for pregnant women, was problematic. Finally, there was absolutely no available treatment for pregnant methamphetamine users.

The Harm Reduction Model

Critics of America's zero-tolerance drug policy advocate a public health orientation to drug problems based on a model of harm reduction (Nadelmann et al. 1994). Proponents of harm reduction accept that overcoming drug addiction is usually a difficult and gradual process. They seek to turn public policy away from punitive criminal justice approaches and toward providing drug abusers with information and assistance that can help them reduce drug consumption and minimize the risks associated with their continuing drug use. Harm reductionists favor drug treatment over imprisonment and favor broadening drug treatment to include non-abstinence–based models.

Although harm-reduction ideas have been more widely accepted in Europe than the United States, certain harm-reduction practices, such as methadone maintenance and needle-exchange programs, are now woven into American drug policy. Harm-reduction programs that specifically target pregnant drug users, however, are practically nonexistent. Moreover, pregnant drug users are often refused admittance into harm-reduction programs created for general population drug users (Sterk 1998). Even committed harm reductionists, it seems, are ambivalent about incorporating pregnant drug users into their model. In general, they define drug use as a victimless crime; however, when it comes to pregnant drug users, the presence of the fetus, as an unwitting participant, causes them to pause. Thus, while harm reductionists object, in principle, to policies that demand abstinence as a condition of offering drug users help and assistance, they have been reluctant to advocate harm-reduction policies for pregnant drug users. The unfortunate irony of this attitude, as this study shows, is that pregnancy often serves as the impetus for women drug users to embrace harm-reduction ideals.

Throughout their pregnancies, PAD Project women engaged in a variety of harm-reduction practices. For the most part, they did so without institutional support and without access to accurate information about prenatal health or the relative dangers of different drug-using practices. A few women sought advice and assistance from social service agencies, drug-treatment programs, and health care providers. Most of the women in our study, however, feared that seeking advice and assistance would trigger institutional interventions of a punitive nature, including forced treatment, imprisonment, and loss of custody of their children. For the most part, women anguished over the potential consequences of their drug use in private; engaged in often uninformed attempts at harm reduction; and hoped against hope that their babies would be born healthy. Labor and delivery in the bright lights of hospital delivery rooms turned private worries into public matters.

5

The Final

Showdown

Birth and
Delivery

Birth was the dénouement—the final showdown in the women's troubled trajectory of drug-involved pregnancy. Constrained by their often economically deprived and chaotic life-styles, women privately acknowledged, continued, or terminated their pregnancies; changed or maintained their drug habits; and attended or avoided prenatal care. Before giving birth, study participants were able to negotiate their lives in relative privacy. The onset of labor, however, changed this immediately and dramatically. Time had run out for women's planned behavioral or life-style changes. By obtaining medical assistance at time of delivery, these pregnant drug users opened themselves up to public scrutiny, which could include legal challenges to their mothering status.

But let us place our interviewees' experiences in the larger social and political context of the late 1980s and early 1990s. Public moral outrage against the pregnant drug user escalated as the media bombarded Americans with vivid

images of drug-damaged babies. Although women of all social classes and ethnic backgrounds use drugs during pregnancy, media stories during this time period overwhelmingly
featured lower-class women of color as users of illegal drugs,
particularly crack cocaine (Humphries 1999, Morgan and
Zimmer 1997, Reinarman and Levine 1997, Sterk 1998).
Medical and social service agencies began monitoring pregnant women more closely for signs of substance use, and in
some states legislatures enacted mandatory reporting protocols for health care providers or punitive sanctions for detected
drug users (McNulty 1987, Paltrow 1992, Siegel 1997).

Particular groups of women (lower-class women of color
versus white middle-class women) and specific types of drug
users (crack smokers versus tobacco smokers) were differentially drug tested and targeted for the more punitive social service and criminal justice interventions (Chasnoff,
Landress, and Barrett 1990; Vega et al. 1993). There were
also important race- and class-based differences in women's
abilities to conceal their drug use during birth and delivery.
Middle-class mothers' drugs of choice were legal—primarily
alcohol and nicotine. They did not carry the same stigma
among health care providers and the general public as the
illegal, so-called harder drugs our interviewees used: heroin,
crack/cocaine, or methamphetamine. The women in our
study believed they were selected for drug testing over the
white middle-class women who delivered babies alongside
them. Testing positive for drug use set in motion a series of
social service and criminal justice interventions that ultimately drove a wedge between women and their role as
mothers.

Why do we as a society reserve our most vitriolic condemnation for pregnant users of illegal drugs? Feminist writers
examining the intractability of the myths enveloping motherhood, particularly the ideology of the entirely nurturant

mother, have found that "in the collision of reality with mythology, it is the mythology that tends to prevail, as the language and the conventions of the story shape not only what is thought but also what can be said, not what is heard but can be understood" (Pope, Quinn, and Wyer 1990, 445). The authors further claim that the "ideology of mothering can be so powerful that the failure of lived experience to validate often produces either intensified efforts to achieve it or a destructive cycle of self- or mother-blame" (442). No other group of mothers lays claim to the unspeakable in quite the same way that pregnant drug users do.

No woman inhabits the all-giving-mother role entirely, but drug-using mothers may miss by the most. Mother as fetal poisoner, or user of illegal drugs, is the antithesis of the prevailing myth of mother as unflagging, unselfish caregiver. Even when women made substantial strides during pregnancy to reduce the risk of drug use to their babies, they discovered at the time of delivery that their lived experiences failed to validate their worth as mothers. In this chapter, we follow women through the public unveiling of their drug use and their continuing efforts to reconcile the conflicting roles of drug user and mother. Throughout, the image of the ideal mythical mother loomed over these women's shoulders and over the shoulders of people with the power to determine their futures. With the onset of labor, women who had not already disclosed faced the immediate dilemma of whether or not to tell the hospital staff about their drug use during pregnancy. Women believed that revealing their drug use might be in the best interest of their babies. But women also knew that revealing their drug use would seriously compromise their claim for custody of their babies. Whichever path they chose, their role as mother would be threatened.

Disclosing versus Concealing Drug Use

Fears and concerns about the baby-to-be's health and insecurity regarding their capacity to be good mothers are problems that plague most pregnant women. Our interviewees' drug use added another layer of fear onto these normal concerns and anxieties. In choosing to disclose or conceal their prenatal drug use, interviewees were forced to confront their two biggest fears: first, because of their drug use, their babies might be born seriously impaired; second, because of their drug use, their babies might be taken away from them.

Veronica's narrative portrays most women's feelings of guilt when they talked about their drug use and its consequences for their babies' health:

> Yeah, after they see the baby come out strung out [withdrawing from drugs], that's the worst. They're gonna feel so bad because that's the way it made me feel. . . . Yeah, it's really hard to live with, and you blame yourself all your life, especially if the baby—something mentally happens to the baby later. You're gonna really blame yourself, which it is our fault for getting high. But that'll always be in your conscience, always in the back of our mind, that it's your fault.

Maya expressed many interviewees' concerns about losing children:

> And then every time I think about doing it, I picture them taking my kids away again, and that would hurt so bad. 'Cause we never been separated unless they went and visit relatives or my daughter went and visited her father or something like that. But other than that, we never been away like this. And seeing them crying and knowing I couldn't do anything about it,

that hurts. And every time I start thinking about it, it started coming up in my mind about crack cocaine. It just—the pictures just flash of them going away again. And that will never happen again, never.

As we detailed in chapter 4, many of our interviewees attempted to reduce fetal harm through drug-use disclosure to prenatal care providers, while at the same time struggling to retain custody of their newborns and older children. As we will see, in labor and delivery wards women's strategies for achieving one purpose often conflicted with achieving the other.

Most pregnant women go to hospitals during labor because they believe it is the best thing to do for themselves and for their babies. Health care providers monitor the progress of labor and help to allay women's fears. For our study participants, the situation was complicated by their own and their health care providers' belief that they must disclose their drug use. In California, as in many other states, drug use during pregnancy can be interpreted as child abuse. If it is so interpreted, hospital staff members are required by law to initiate child protection or law enforcement referrals.[1] Thus, if women revealed their drug use, they risked losing custody of their newborns as well as their older children. Ironically, strategies to alleviate drug-related fetal damage (drug-use disclosure) exacerbated the likelihood of the other predominate maternal fear: Child Protective Service interventions.

Whether or not to disclose drug use to health care workers was a topic of serious concern for PAD participants. The women's decisions to disclose or conceal were often well-thought-out strategies implemented to attempt to accomplish their two main objectives: a healthier baby and maternal custody. Although women expected that disclosure would improve their newborns' care, at the same time they risked exposing themselves to CPS interventions. Despite these risks, many women openly disclosed their use to health care providers. Other women, who shared these same maternal goals, chose to conceal their drug use.

Disclosing

The most important difference between disclosers and concealers was women's perceptions of the providers' capabilities to mitigate the effects of illicit drug use. For those women who disclosed, fear of newborn morbidity overrode fears of custody loss. Disclosers saw providers as helpers. For them, the first step toward enlisting complete cooperation and assistance was to reveal their drug use. Amanda's account typified this strategic response: "Please don't let nothing happen to my baby. I don't want nothing to happen to him. God, please. I will tell my doctor, I will tell her, 'Is my baby gonna be okay? Please help me.'"

Disclosing drug use was Amanda's strategy for not letting anything happen to her baby. Like other disclosers, she assumed that her provider's medical expertise and available techniques could palliate the effects of her drug use.

Medical help had a variety of meanings for women. Hospital providers offered referrals to parenting programs, drug-treatment programs, useful health information, and links to social services. For these women, revealing their drug problems was a way to tap into these resources.

Some disclosers sought to capitalize on what they perceived to be the advanced obstetrical technology necessary to mitigate the effects of their drug use. At the time of delivery, these women viewed sonograms, fetal monitors, IVs, incubators, medications, and other medical procedures as interventions that could help their babies survive their drug use. While women could not erase the times in which they had used drugs, many found comfort in the chance to hear the baby's heartbeat and confirm through fetal monitors that their labor was progressing normally. Drug-use disclosure was a way to ensure that all possible precautions were taken and medical interventions implemented.

Once women were identified as drug users, social structural or institutional forces came into play. The women's attempts to receive better care through technological intervention were sometimes undermined by the ramifications of being identified as a drug-using mother.

Once women were publicly identified, they were often stigmatized by labor and delivery staff. Clara, a white thirty-two-year-old heroin user, explained why she failed to visit her child in the nursery:

> I didn't go one day to see him at the hospital because . . .
> I don't know if you know what nurses are like, but especially at [a public hospital] they literally stood there and said, "Your baby's sick and you did it to your baby. . . . We have really sick babies to take care of, and you did this to your child." You know, but who could sit there for twelve hours a day with these nurses and their really negative attitudes?

Some women were not prepared to face the anger and outrage that disclosures sometimes precipitated. Even the women who managed to quit using in the weeks or months before delivery reported that they were treated badly despite their attempts. Mariah explained her frustration in trying to convince hospital personnel that she had stopped using drugs three months before: "They were asking me all—oooh, they were asking me every minute. I said, 'I told you I'm not on drugs no more. I used to use drugs like twelve weeks ago.' I said, 'But I'm not on drugs no more.'"

Women reported that health care providers were quick to assume that drug users would lie about their use. Heather's experience indicates some providers' distrust and lack of information regarding drug use:

Interviewer: How did they treat you?
Heather: Like shit. They—we'd had an outbreak of body lice a week before. We spent a hundred dollars on laundry, cleaning up that apartment getting ready for this baby to come. . . . Well, I had scars like, bites all over my body. They're saying that I displayed track marks all over my body. I told them, "Sure, all over my belly. All over my legs. Come on."

After disclosing, the women were frustrated by providers' suspicion, distrust, and misinformation about drug use. The women also noted that many caregivers became watchful and wary of their subsequent behaviors.

Concealing

A few study participants, anticipating the potential for emotional trauma attached to disclosing, opted for concealment strategies. Some women went to labor and delivery but were adamant about not letting their caregivers know about their drug use.

For these women, concealing meant forgoing care all together and planning to have children outside hospital settings. "Being up in their business" or violations of privacy were concerns for them. These interviewees had strong convictions that information about drug use was personal and should remain inaccessible to medical personnel.

Naomi recounted why she would never tell the truth about her heroin use in a health care setting again: "I was also discriminated against . . . because I told the truth. They asked me about my [drug-use] history . . . the day I was supposed to go in, called me up and said, 'I'm sorry, but we can't help you because of your history of IV use.'"

Other concealers did more than simply refuse to tell the truth. Some women wanted to avoid traditional health care settings all together. Julia explained her method for accessing needed medical information:

> *Julia:* I talked to doctors on the phone. Because if you talk to people face to face, then they get into that technicality about child abuse. . . . I called University of California and Stanford and every main hospital I could think of to talk to them.
>
> *Interviewer:* And what were the—and you felt comfortable asking any question over the phone?
>
> *Julia:* Right, it was anonymous. The thing that they said that might happen would be a cleft lip, which I really wasn't even sure what that was but I said, "Okay."

By remaining anonymous and asking questions over the phone, Julia was able to alleviate some of her concerns without exposing herself or her child to what she believed were the recriminations of identification as a pregnant drug user.

Concealers were very similar to disclosers in their concerns and goals. The main difference between the two groups was how they evaluated their chances of meeting their objectives in traditional health care settings. Disclosers felt that providers would help them improve their babies' health and that because of their cooperation they would keep custody of their children. Concealers did not believe that providers would help them achieve their goals. They were more likely to believe that caregivers would condemn or penalize them for their drug use during pregnancy.

Drug Testing: Hospital Practices and Policies

Whether or not women disclosed their drug use during prenatal care visits or at the time of delivery, if they used illegal drugs in the two to four days before the birth, drug tests of maternal and newborn urine would document heroin, crack/cocaine, or methamphetamine use. Some PAD participants thought that only women and their infants who fit hospital profiles of typical street-drug users were tested for drugs. Most interviewees, however, believed that if a pregnant woman of color presented for delivery in a San Francisco Bay Area hospital, she and her baby would be automatically tested for drug use.

We did not discover any uniform policy for the drug testing of mothers and infants. Nevertheless, the pediatric social workers we interviewed claimed that every hospital in the Bay Area had devised drug-testing protocols, such as written memos; word-of-mouth guidelines; and special instructions designed to train hospital staff to detect, test, and report cases of maternal drug use. Generally, the profile of women and babies targeted for testing included women who had failed to get consistent prenatal care, admitted to using drugs in the past, appeared to be intoxicated at the time of delivery, or had lost custody of their older children.

Most women believed that birth was the time when they most likely would be tested for drug use. Often, their image of drug-testing protocols differed from actual hospital policies and practices. For example, Sasha contended that she could not avoid being tested upon giving birth: "Do you know that in California they automatically test you if you're a woman of color? . . . It's true. If you're white, they won't test you unless you have a history [with drugs]. . . . Yeah, if you're Mexican or black, they automatically [snaps fingers]. Even the Catholic hospitals."

Like Sasha, other women felt they would be tested for

drugs, no matter what. Jackie never tried to hide her drug use from the labor and delivery room nurses or doctors because she felt they knew about her crack use because they took her urine specimen: "They all know. It was like no secret. I wasn't trying to hide it, 'cause soon as they took my urine, they was gonna know anyway."

Since we did not have access to Jackie's medical records, we do not know whether her urine was taken for a toxicological screening or for some other type of test. During the time when our interviewees were giving birth, drug-testing protocols were anything but uniform. In most health care settings, whether or not a woman was tested was a staff decision. Nonetheless, regardless of whether the women and their newborns were actually uniformly or selectively drug tested, women's perceptions of hospital practices influenced their behaviors and escalated their anxieties.

The Unveiling

An important dimension of the final showdown was the unveiling—the moment when the women were forced to confront their previously private fears. It was also a public moment, when delivery-room staff evaluated a newborn's health, interpreted the possible causes of any negative outcomes, and decided whether to initiate institutional responses.

Fears

The women's fears of physiological problems resulting from their drug use were often dramatic and ranged from loss of limbs to extra body parts to malformation of major organs. Few women reported concern about the most common reported outcomes of heroin-, cocaine-, and methamphetamine-involved pregnancies: prematurity, lowered birth weight, and smaller head circumference (Acker et al. 1983; Chasnoff et al. 1985; Chasnoff 1988; Finnegan 1988; Habel, Kaye, and Lee 1990; Naeye et al. 1973; Pettiti and Coleman 1990; Racine, Joyce, and Anderson 1993; Wilson et al. 1979). Naomi and Kristen outlined their fears about how the drugs they used might affect their babies.

> *Naomi:* Look, I've shot speed. I've shot heroin, and I'm afraid I'm going to have a baby with fifty thousand fingers and eight thousand eyeballs.

> *Kristen:* Maybe my baby might come out with two fingers. You never know. Or might just be born stillborn.

Another important source of women's apprehensions about their newborn outcomes was the considerable media attention given to the issue of maternal drug use in the late 1980s and early 1990s. The actual connection between media coverage and consequent individual perceptions of drug effects on the unborn and on pregnant women's behavior is beyond the scope of the present research and needs more thorough investigation. Nevertheless, the media's portrayal of in-utero drug exposure was widespread and often exaggerated (Humphries 1999). According to numerous media stories, children exposed to cocaine in utero would either die or be dangerously impaired. In such portrayals, there was no chance for children exposed to cocaine in utero to ever enjoy normal lives. In this political climate, it was no wonder that our interviewees often braced themselves for the worst.

Another source of women's fears was the accounts of other drug-using mothers' experiences of newborn morbidity and mortality. Darleen reported: "My friend . . . who just had a baby with the two holes in his heart . . . she was getting high [smoking crack], right, when she had it. She went into labor as she was getting high."

Evania talked about her nephew who was exposed to crack in utero: "Yeah, he lived for about a year after getting out of the hospital. He was in the hospital for like eight months. And I think when he turned a year, he got a foster parent and stuff and they moved him out to Oakland. And then he was only, I think he was right about a year old and he died. His lungs just collapsed."

As Darleen's and Evania's stories suggest, most women believed that their drug use would lead to negative newborn outcomes. Women told us that tales of others' bad experiences influenced their feelings about their own pregnancies.

Previous drug-involved pregnancies also influenced the women's ideas about potential outcomes, and babies with drug-related problems at birth confirmed the mothers' fears. Even if the babies did not have problems at birth, women still worried. At time of interview, Kristen was fifteen weeks' pregnant and had quit smoking crack for what she hoped would be the duration of her pregnancy. Unfortunately, she had not been able to quit during her previous pregnancy. Her four-year-old daughter was born prematurely and weighed just three pounds. Kristen was very worried before, during, and after the birth. She regretted her drug use even though her daughter's weight and size soon caught up with other babies her age.

Looking back on this experience, Kristen felt that God had granted her a healthy baby despite her drug use. With her current pregnancy, she did not want to depend on God's continued intervention, "'cause maybe this time God is not gonna grant me the satisfaction to say, 'Oh, yeah, my baby's healthy.'"

During labor and delivery, many women reported praying to a higher power to intervene and allow their children to emerge unscathed from in-utero drug exposure. According to these women's perspectives, their baby's outcome was now in the hands of powers such as fate or God.

Birth was when women were forced to confront their persistent fears and witness firsthand the consequences of their drug use during pregnancy. Time had run out for pregnancy-long plans to discontinue drug use or to adhere to healthy regimens. The women's descriptions were akin to biblical depictions of the final judgment day, when good deeds, such as efforts to improve health, were weighed against bad deeds, such as continuing to use drugs or failing to keep prenatal care appointments.

Infant Health Problems

Before describing women's reports about their babies' health at birth, we must restate some methodological caveats. Due to the nature of our sampling techniques and methods of data collection, we cannot generalize from our findings about actual incidence or prevalence of drug-related problems associated with drug-involved pregnancies. To recruit study participants, we posted flyers in public places (described in more detail in the appendix). The first line of our flyer read, "Women Drug Users: Are you pregnant or do you have an infant?" By advertising for pregnant women or women with infants, we may have inadvertently excluded drug users whose children had died or were severely ill. Additionally, guilt and grief may have kept such women from participating in our study and recounting their emotional trauma to strangers. Finally, we relied solely on women's self-reports of physicians' evaluations of their infants' health. Due to the stigma associated with drug use during pregnancy, some women may have tended to underreport problems or to downplay their severity.

Nonetheless, thirty-five of the forty women who had

given birth by the time of interview reported that their newborns experienced problems at birth. There were no stillborns and no reports of serious deformities, malformations, or complications. However, 20 percent of the women (eight) gave birth prematurely (from three to thirteen weeks before their projected due date), 27 percent (eleven) reported that their children were born with some medical complications, and 40 percent (sixteen) reported that their newborns experienced withdrawal symptoms.

The medical complications included click hips, jaundice, meconium staining, extra skin tags on infants' hands, lethargy, poor eating, poor weight gain, and a cleft lip. While nearly half of the women claimed that their infants experienced withdrawal, the severity of withdrawal symptoms ranged from reports of general irritability and sleeplessness for one night to diarrhea, sweating, and shaking for several weeks. Two of the women (5 percent) did not observe withdrawal symptoms themselves but were told by hospital staff that their newborns had suffered from drug withdrawal in the nursery. Most women who reported premature birth, infant medical complications, and withdrawal symptoms reported *mild* symptoms and conditions.

These data suggest that women's experiences, while not always positive, were not as frightening as they had expected. The newborns of the forty women who had recently given birth were not the picture of health, but they did not mirror the then popular media depictions of a permanently doomed generation.

Relief

Many women were, for the most part, pleasantly surprised and extremely relieved to find that their children were born with all their limbs and, more often than not, within the range of normal weights and lengths and with all of their internal organs intact. Veronica recalled her unexpected joy at delivering a healthy baby boy: "He was the smartest thing there was, that little kid. He was so smart. And he didn't go through any withdrawals or anything. I know it doesn't sound right to be bragging about it, but I was even shocked because I expected the worst."

Continuing Guilt

While our findings indicate that many women did not confront problems as severe as they had imagined during pregnancy, interviewees were not absolved from guilt after birth. The guilt of using drugs during pregnancy persisted even when their children experienced few, if any, problems. For example, Bronwen, a thirty-five-year-old African-American crack smoker, felt guilty about her drug use during pregnancy and worried about what was happening to her baby in utero. She explained that she had planned to have an abortion in the beginning of her pregnancy, so she continued to use crack. As the pregnancy progressed, she found it increasingly difficult to go through with the abortion and eventually decided not to terminate the pregnancy. Looking back at her use in the beginning of the pregnancy, she became very concerned about the possible problems she had caused by failing to abstain. She told us about her guilt:

> The guilt, being like four months' pregnant and still using and the baby still moving, and I had no idea whether that was the baby having spasms or having a heart attack. And I was just like scared to death. . . . Yes, feeling the movement but still, at the same time, not knowing if it was moving because of life or if it was moving because of a heart attack or whatever.

As Bronwen's due date approached, her apprehension escalated. Although her health care providers tried to reassure her through routine checks and sonograms that her pregnancy was progressing normally, she continued to worry. The birth itself was fraught with even more guilt and anxiety. She depicted her emotional state in the weeks before the birth and during delivery:

> *Bronwen:* It was real scary because of the anticipation. I was given a due date of June twenty-eighth and he didn't come until August first . . . and, well, I just knew that it was my fault. So they were trying to keep me unstressful and to remain calm, and I had like all of the tests that could be taken, the amnio and sonograms once a month. So they finally had me reassured. During labor—I went in something like 9:00 that morning. At 7:00 that evening, he was born. But I was in a lot of pain, and I was determined not to take any drug. . . . And it's like, "Oh, my God, I'm doing this by myself." And it was like five pushes and he still hadn't come. And I'm, "I can't do this any more." And they're going, "Yes, you can." And I go, "No, I can't." "One more, one more." And I push him out and he's blue, and they call, "Get the nursery down here, stat." And I go, "Oh, my God, what's wrong with him?" And from the position that I was in and where they had the baby, all I could see was these little tabs of fat hanging. That was from the extra digits. . . . They took him away and about an hour later, they brought him back and by this time, he had made it here and I felt really relieved.
>
> *Interviewer:* What happened in that hour? Did they not tell you anything?
>
> *Bronwen:* Oh, yeah. They told me, "Well, he's fine." But they wanted to monitor him and take his vitals and clean him up. And so, yeah. But once I made it back into my bed where I was gonna be at, they brought him in to me and it's like I just broke down in tears. I think a lot of it was from joy to

see that he was okay, glad that it was over with,
and it was a mixed combination of everything.

As Bronwen's story illustrates, birth was a time of complex and sometimes conflicting emotions when women felt
relief and sorrow, excitement and worry. Bronwen was relieved that her son was healthy, and the doctors reassured
her that he was fine. Nonetheless, she could not help but
feel anxious about the delay of the birth and the skin tags
on her son's hands. Later, when asked about her son's health
and her birth experiences, she told us that she believed
the skin tags were probably caused by her drug use during
pregnancy.

Ethel gave birth to a son, who was also born without
apparent complications or withdrawals. During the first four
months of pregnancy, she was not able to stop smoking
crack, although pregnancy made her panic about her child's
future. She recalled her emotional breakdown due to remorse
after giving birth:

You know, I was using and this little baby was suffering and *I was using.* And he had—I mean, it's like this
little, little thing. It's like, "How could you do that to
him?" It was so sad. And I had told God—I still feel
bad about that, but I had told God to help me with this
'cause it was like I had asked him to give me a baby
when he thought I was ready and so I must be ready
because I have my baby. And I asked them to take the
test to see if they were toxic and—if he was toxic—
and the test came back negative, and I was like, "Yes!"
And K. [her social worker] had told me she would give
it to me, and it was just like, "Oh, my God, this is my
baby!" It was—oh, it was so emotional! And at 3:00 in
the morning, I called the nurse and I was like, "I want
my baby," and I just held him. He was sleeping, and I

held him and I cried and I just kept saying over and over again, "I'm so sorry. I didn't know what I was doing." And I promised to him that I was gonna do the best that I can, to be the best mom that I can be. And that's what I'm doing today is the best that I can for today. But it was really hard. That was like the hardest part was to see my baby and then know what I was doing.

As these women's narratives suggest, regardless of the outcome of the unveiling, their regret and guilt often persisted.

Birth, and the multiple emotions that usually accompanied this life-transforming event, was often complicated by interviewees' heightened concerns for their children's health. Even positive newborn outcomes did not absolve the women from the guilt resulting from their drug use and its effects on their children's health and well-being. Women noted that children were not as damaged as they expected, and many of our interviewees reported no drug-related problems. As Ethel's story suggests, staring into a newborn's tiny face often reminded women of what they had risked by using drugs while pregnant.

Battling the Baby Snatchers

The other dimension of the final showdown was, as one woman characterized it, "battling the baby snatchers." Birth was the dangerous window of time when women's continued custody of their children was most at risk.

Child Protective Services interventions into mothers' and newborns' lives were neither certain nor uniform. While many of the women believed that being drug tested during labor and delivery was guaranteed, they viewed CPS interventions as much more arbitrary. From PAD participants' perspectives, there was no clear pattern as to which mothers hospital staff would refer to CPS and, once referred, which kinds of maternal-newborn circumstances would result in loss of custody. The possibility of confronting positive drug tests was difficult and traumatic for women. The anticipation of losing custody, on the other hand, was devastating. Interviewees were somewhat like Californians anticipating an earthquake. They knew it could happen but hoped and often prayed such a tragedy would not visit their lives. To illustrate the different outcomes of CPS interventions and their effect on women's lives, we present the following three accounts. Marilyn invited her interviewer into her home with open arms. She made caring for her sleeping newborn and her two-and-a-half-year-old son, whom she called "Little Man," look amazingly easy while she candidly told her story in the course of our lengthy interview.

Her pregnancy with Little Man was much more difficult than her pregnancy with her newborn. Throughout her son's pregnancy, she attempted to manage a full-time job and a full-time crack addiction. In the third month of pregnancy, she lost her job, went on unemployment, and continued smoking crack until the birth. During the sixth month, she went into premature labor and gave birth to Little Man, whom the doctors told her would never walk or talk. She described her reactions:

> It was like, "That's a baby?" She said, "This is your baby." "That's my baby?" By this time, my son had his face bruised, you know, was dark, real dark and his body was colored here. And I'm like, "Well, how in the hell did I do that? How did I give birth to a two-toned baby?" It looked like a little frog. It had all these little needles and shit sticking out, all those catheters on top of his head . . . but he had all his fingers and his toes . . . and she [the nurse] said, "You are lucky. You are really lucky." And I'm like, "Wow! This is a baby."

At the same time that Marilyn faced the tenuous nature of Little Man's health, she also faced losing her right to mother him since they had both tested positive for cocaine. Marilyn talked about managing her CPS intervention along with her son's frail health:

> I'm not kidding. I tried to lie [about her drug use during pregnancy]. . . . I had to deal with that shit [a custody case]. I didn't know nothing about them people [CPS social workers]. He [her social worker] was a nice person. He was a nice guy. And being that my son stayed in the hospital for four and a half months, I know they was going to have to have somebody come out to my house. He would have these people call me. But he [her son] stayed in the hospital, see. I was there at the hospital every day, all day long, shit like that. I remember the lady told me because I know I really fucked up. But I loved my son, and it was something that I did that was having him going through the shit that he went through. And I beat myself up. I loved my son, and I knew I had to deal with whatever was going to be, you know, whether he be handicapped or whatever. I would be glad to deal with it. . . . If I hadn't been there for my son, he probably wouldn't be here today, you know. And I was there for a month.

Later in her interview, she recounted her experience with her CPS worker:

> I had those people [the hospital staff] give me a place in this building . . . across the street. It was part of the hospital where the resident doctors stayed . . . was my house, you know. 'Cause I wasn't leaving my son. So I did all my—I did all that time in there for them CPS. That's when I seen that CPS person one time. After

that, I took my son home. One time and I didn't see her no more after that. . . . She came and closed the book, you know, 'cause I had been at the hospital, and what I was supposed to do at the hospital? Nobody told me that's what I had to do. See, that's what I had to do for me. I didn't have anybody telling me what to do.

From Marilyn's perspective, the custody battle was secondary to the struggle to save her son's life. Social workers and impending custody hearings faded into the background as she put all her energy into improving her son's health. After she was able to take her son home, and after just one visit from the CPS worker, she was granted custody. Marilyn's interpretation of this decision was "'cause I had been at the hospital," but no one from hospital staff or CPS had instructed her about how to increase her chances of retaining custody. When we interviewed Marilyn, Little Man was a typical curious and rambunctious two-year-old who kept both Marilyn and the interviewer on their toes, climbing all over both of them and asking countless questions.

Other women's accounts of CPS interventions were quite different from Marilyn's. Abigail had an exceedingly difficult time trying to keep custody of her newborn daughter. After the birth, her daughter suffered some methadone withdrawal and tested positive for both methadone and heroin. Abigail explained her heroin use:

I did do dope like three or four days before the baby was born 'cause I thought I still had two more months to go, but that's still no excuse. So the tests came up dirty, which scared me to death because mostly— usually when your test comes up dirty, there's no questions. They're gonna take your baby away, and you have to try and get it back.

In Abigail's situation, the fight for custody was a battle between two opposing forces. One was her social worker, the other her doctor. Abigail described their opposing positions:

> I consider myself really lucky, but my social worker saw something else in me where she believed—she kind of in a way worked towards helping me keep my baby rather than it being taken away. But there was nothing that was gonna change the other doctor's mind at all. Whether I came up dirty or not, because the fact that the baby was on methadone, and the way I looked and my mother looked, she just—we weren't like—we were all wrong for this baby. This poor little baby was gonna have this horrible life. And she [the doctor] accused me of lying.

As Abigail's narrative suggests, the battle for custody was often an unknown and apparently arbitrary event. CPS workers, nurses, doctors, and hospital social workers could either act as a mother's advocate in her efforts to ensure family unity or take the role of the child's advocate and work toward removing the child from the "unfit" mother's home. Abigail's custody case included both interventional styles. She claimed that her doctor tried to paint a picture of her as a poor parent while she was in the hospital and all during her daughter's nineteen days in the hospital nursery. Since the final decision was in the hands of the CPS social worker, Abigail retained custody of her daughter despite her doctor's objections.

Sally lost custody of her newborn daughter. Sally's periods had never been regular, and she did not confirm her pregnancy until the week before giving birth. Sally used methamphetamine three times a week during her pregnancy but was planning to quit in the near future. Unfortunately, before she had the chance to quit using, she went into premature labor and gave birth to a four-pound, eleven-ounce baby girl. Both she and the baby's father were distraught over their continued methamphetamine use. Sally explained to the hospital staff and CPS workers that she and the baby's father did not realize that she was in her third trimester. Sally recalled her delayed discovery of pregnancy and early delivery:

> I was gonna go in and have a pregnancy test then just virtually so I could go in and get Medi-Cal and everything else. And we [Sally and the baby's father] figured I was only a few months' pregnant. And it turned out, "Oh, and here she is!" And I knew I was pregnant, but we thought I was only like the first couple months' pregnant. We felt real bad about it [using drugs during pregnancy], but it was like we didn't realize I was that far along. It wasn't anything that was done really intentionally. We had plans on taking—we were trying to get the money together to get a vehicle so that we didn't have to ride the bus back to Maryland. But we wanted to go back to Maryland to his [the baby's father] mom's before we had the baby so that we were away from the drugs and could have the baby and everything else. And then maybe the state wouldn't bother us and we could have everything taken care of all at once. So it was like then the next thing we knew, I had her. But we had every intention of leaving and getting out of the drug scene. And we didn't realize that I was as far as I was, and we sure didn't expect her to be two, two and a half months early.

Sally and her husband tried to get on the nurses' and doctors' good side while in the hospital in an attempt to improve their chances of parenting their daughter. Without being asked, they told the doctors how many drugs they both had used during the pregnancy. Both she and her husband kept every appointment with social workers and health care providers and visited their daughter regularly.

According to Sally, her interactions with providers and CPS workers did not go well. She said that CPS workers, nurses, and doctors told her that "everything was on account of the drugs." She tried to explain why she did not get prenatal care or quit using drugs, but she was never able to convince them that she was a capable parent or that she had honestly planned to quit using. Sally remembered how she learned that she had lost custody of her baby girl:

> *Sally:* The Social Services court got custody of her.
> *Interviewer:* Because they tested her for drugs and they said that's what . . . ?
> *Sally:* Yeah, which we knew. They didn't have to do the drug test. We already told them the drugs were there. "Well, the baby tested positive with drugs in her." "Yeah, well, we kinda told you that before the baby was ever here to test. What more do you want?" And so then how long did she spend in the hospital? Let's see, she was there for about a week, and then they finally—as a matter of fact, we'd gone to court and they said, "Go up and see the baby when you get out of the court," with my attorney and his attorney. Well, we had enough bus fare for one of us, but we had a bicycle, too. It was still at Hillsdale. And [my husband] says, "You go and ride the bus, and I'll ride the bike up and meet you there." Well, I got to the hospital and walked into the nursery and couldn't find [the baby]. So I walked in to see the nurse to find out where [the baby] is 'cause they were cleaning up the nursery, so I figured they might have moved her again 'cause they'd done that the day before. And finally, they sent the doctor out and he says, "Well, she's been moved." And I says, "What do

you mean she's been moved?" He went, "Children's Services Division came and took her to a foster home." And I lost it.

Unlike Marilyn and Abigail, Sally was not able to convince the authorities that she could parent adequately or provide a suitable home environment.

Relying solely on these women's accounts, we find a lack of uniformity in CPS intervention outcomes. All three women had used drugs in the week before delivery, all three newborns experienced symptoms associated with drug-involved pregnancies, each had failed to get consistent pre-natal care, each had problematic housing arrangements, and only one (who lost custody) had the participation of the child's father during their custody review process.

Sally, unlike the other two women, had lost custody of children in the past. This may or may not have weighed more heavily against her. Marilyn lied about her drug use to everyone involved and told them she had smoked a cigarette that might have been laced with cocaine. This may have helped her case. Finally, Abigail's mother became very active during the custody review process and promised to help Abigail raise the child. There may be numerous other reasons that explain these three women's differing encounters with CPS, such as the availability of foster care, CPS workers' caseloads, or differences in hospital protocols. From the women's perspective, custody interventions appeared to be arbitrary, discretionary, and ultimately terrifying.

For the most part, our interviewees believed that CPS cases were not based on a strict formula or a protocol that was evenly or fairly administered. PAD study participants believed that the decision to refer women and babies to CPS and the entire intervention process was subjective and based upon potentially biased interpretations of hospital staff, social workers, and CPS workers. Like protocols for testing mothers and infants for drug use in labor and delivery wards, the manner in which women were selected to be reported to CPS may have differed from health care provider to health care provider. Likewise, the evaluative factors for custody determinations may have varied from CPS worker to CPS worker.

According to Abigail, her doctor saw her as an unfit mother while her social worker considered her a vulnerable mother in need of family support services. If Abigail's social worker had agreed with her doctor, her custody outcome may have looked more like Sally's. Attempting to comply and work within such a framework made dealing with the CPS intervention process as difficult as predicting newborns' health problems. Whether a child emerged from in-utero drug exposure unaffected appeared to our interviewees to be almost as arbitrary and subject to whim, fate, or divine intervention. So, too, was the retention or loss of custody of their infants. Finally, for the women who lost the battle with the baby snatchers, their universal response was to go on an extended drug-using binge to dim their memories and drown their sorrows.

The public unveiling of infants' outcomes forced these women to face previously private fears in very public settings. Births were laced with powerful and mixed emotions that were often compounded by heightened concerns about babies' health. Even positive newborn outcomes did not absolve women from feelings of guilt derived from their drug use during pregnancy. While interviewees celebrated, thanking God or invoking the fates when children were not as damaged as they expected, they still worried about, and felt responsible for, problems that might arise in the future.

The second, and equally problematic, dimension of the final showdown was battling the baby snatchers. From our interviewees' perspective, CPS referrals and the consequences of interventions were for the most part arbitrary and discretionary and beyond women's ability to predict or control. The women who retained custody began their mothering careers by failing. They failed to fulfill the most basic part of the good mother myth: mother as nurturer. Not only did most of them believe that they had failed to eat and sleep properly during pregnancy, they also introduced poisons into their helpless infants' systems before they were even born. They returned to the neighborhoods and relationships in which they had continued to use drugs while pregnant and tried to stay sober while caring night and day for a sometimes sickly infant.

Those women who lost custody of their infants at birth usually spiraled downward into drug-fueled destructive cycles of self-blame. These women lost not only their children but yet another opportunity to inhabit a positive and productive social role. With the number of accessible, available, and respectable social positions shrinking with each passing year, getting pregnant again and again while trying each time to become a "good" mother became one available lifeline.

6

"Not Good

Enough to

Be Pregnant"

Conclusions
and Policy
Implications

Many of our interviewees were victimized and brutalized almost from birth. Basics, such as their right to control their own bodies, were violated through incest, molestation, rape, and battering. Some women were removed from family homes due to violence or abuse and then abused and violated in subsequent settings. Unsafe and unstable home environments pushed women out of family homes in early or late adolescence. These women were then faced with a myriad of problems resulting from racism, poverty, teenage pregnancy, lack of education, and chronic unemployment. When they worked, they were segregated into primarily monotonous, menial, and minimum-wage jobs. Then drugs came into their lives. With these terrible traumas and limited resources, women faced the prospect of motherhood.

As we have discussed, the discovery period was characterized by ambivalence. Women identified body changes, ascribing them to or denying them as symptoms of pregnancy. This stage could last from a few weeks to several months or more, during which women would privately alternate between admitting and denying being pregnant. We called this time the beginning of the private dilemma because a public discussion (even with the father) was tantamount to acceptance of the impending birth. Public expression of a woman's suspicions usually meant that her significant others would insist she get some concrete confirmation (a pregnancy test) or begin interacting with her as a mother-to-be.

This private dilemma had implications for maternal and fetal health. It was complicated by the social, familial, moral, economic, and emotional issues that surrounded decisions to abort or continue pregnancies. These issues (often in conflict with each other) prolonged the discovery period and exacerbated the difficulty of effective educational, medical, and familial support or interventions. Women could not go to prenatal care or abortion services, even if they were accessible, if they had not accepted or announced their pregnancy. Most women were reticent about going to prenatal care, especially if they believed they would be stigmatized.

There were numerous reasons for this ambivalence. Many women both wanted and did not want to be pregnant. Children were an expensive and long-term commitment. For many women, pregnancy would result in deepening or sometimes initial commitment to their relationship with the father. (This could be a pro or a con.) Pregnancy also had a significant emotional component for most

women. They expected to receive love from the baby—
"someone of my own to love." Love from the father was
also an issue—"if I give him a baby, our love will grow stron-
ger and more solid."

Drug-using women had to deal with another powerful
source of ambivalence. Acceptance or announcement of
pregnancy meant that they (and most others) believed they
should stop all drug and alcohol use immediately. Drug use
was a form of recreation and also helped them to cope with
emotional and physical problems stemming from the vic-
timizations and traumas that most had endured since early
childhood. For some women, the belief that their drug use
had already damaged the developing fetus provided an acceptable rationale for terminating pregnancies. For others,
denial of pregnancy was a way to have it both ways because
they wanted the baby but also wanted to continue using
drugs.

Many women changed their drug-use patterns (types of
drugs used, routes of administration) but were unable to
completely discontinue using. Despite considerable difficulties, both practical (access to scientific literature) and
ideological (generalized beliefs that drug-exposed pregnancies are so compromised that harm reduction is futile), the
women did construct harm-reduction strategies. These included drug switching, reductions in use, changes in routes
of administration, and increased concern about proper nutrition and regular sleeping patterns. In addition to drug effects, some women believed that potential loss of custody
was a major harm to be avoided. Thus, they used folk rem-
edies to avoid urinalysis detection. (Goldenseal and cran-
berry juice were reputed to flush drugs out of their systems.)
Even if they reduced or stopped using, any drugs used while
pregnant were a constant source of guilt and worry. This

colored their initiation into mothering and plagued most women's consciences throughout the pregnancy into the postpartum period.

Pregnancy increased women's responsibilities. A woman was now responsible for the effects and consequences of her drug use on her unborn baby. During pregnancy, protecting the baby's well-being included eating and sleeping regularly and seeking prenatal care. The pregnant woman was now forced to decide whether or not to stay away from or lie to prenatal care providers. Disclosure of drug use to health or social service providers could result in loss of custody. Women balanced their babies' health needs with the risk of not being able to raise the babies themselves. They struggled with this question: in the long term was it better for the baby to tell or not to tell?

Birth was the final showdown, the end of the troubled trajectory of their pregnancies. An important component of the final showdown was the unveiling, the moment when women confronted their previously private fears and the baby was born. It was also a public moment, when delivery-room staff evaluated the newborn's health, interpreted the possible causes of any negative outcomes, and decided whether to initiate institutional responses. Birth, and the multiple emotions that usually accompany this life-transforming event, were often complicated by interviewees' heightened concerns for children's health. Even positive newborn outcomes did not absolve women from the guilt resulting from their drug use and its effects on their children's health and well-being. Some women noted that children were not as damaged as they expected, and some reported no drug-related problems.

The other dimension of the final showdown was "battling the baby snatchers" since birth was the time when continued custody of children was most imperiled. Women who retained custody began their mothering careers by failing because they used drugs during pregnancy and endangered their children. Women who lost custody of their infants usually began abusing their drugs of choice immediately, surpassing previous heavy use by trying to drown painful guilt and self-blame.

Despite lifelong gender-, race-, and class-based subjugation and stigmatizing drug use, study participants implemented strategies to reduce fetal harm and claim respectable social identities. These private struggles were embedded in a socioeconomic context characterized by increasing degradation and deprivation and decreasing social support.

We must place mothering in its historical and political framework to understand its importance for a women's sense of self and social position. It is also necessary for us to explicate the policy context in which our study participants began or postponed motherhood. Finally, we must propose the sorts of social services and support that might better serve both pregnant drug users and their children in light of our findings.

The Political Economy of American Mothering

Mothering is a social role with tremendous responsibilities, little preparation, and ambiguous standards of good practice. People do not necessarily know how to tell a woman to mother, but everybody seems to know when she is doing it wrong. Being labeled an unfit mother has horrendous consequences of personal and social condemnation and social isolation.

Psychoanalyst Estella Welldon (1988) described the difficulties that mothering presents for women:

Women are expected to carry out the difficult and responsible task of motherhood without having had much, if any, emotional preparation for it. Their responsibility is to bring up healthy and stable babies who will adapt happily to growing external demands. In fact, women really are in too lonely a position to deliver the goods properly, and this marks a fundamental difference between men and women. . . . Mothers are expected by society to behave as if they had been provided with magic wands which not only free them from previous conflicts, but also equip them to deal with the new emergencies of motherhood with skill, precision, and dexterity. (1988, 17–18)

With all its loneliness, difficulty, and ambiguity, becoming a mother continues to be the means by which many women achieve full adult status and demonstrate their feminine identity (Chodorow 1978, Notman and Nadelson 1982, Oakley 1980, Salmon 1985).[1] Although the past fifty years have brought enormous changes in women's participation in the paid labor market, women continue to be defined in terms of their reproductive functions. Thus, failure to properly perform mothering responsibilities is tantamount to failure as a woman.

Our interviewees' mothering standards and values resonated with those of most American mothers: mothers should protect their children from harm; keep them fed, warm, presentably dressed, and clean; and see that they are educated, prepared for the work world, and shown right from wrong. These goals are a tall order, however, under conditions of lifelong victimization; lack of skills and education; unplanned childbearing; single parenting; violent and unsafe housing; and scarcity of resources not only for children's play and learning but for basics such as food, clothing, and shelter.

The social construction of adequate mothering must be analyzed in its historical, political, and economic contexts. The social relations through which women's social and economic subordination is perpetuated are predicated upon the gendered division of labor. Feminist theorists link hegemonic idealization of motherhood to the industrial family ethic or the family wage (Abramovitz 1988, Pascall 1986, Quadagno 1987). The family wage refers to the outdated economic and social arrangement in which men are breadwinners and women unpaid homemakers. The persistence of the ideology of a family wage is central to an understanding of a woman as the natural rather than socially constructed child nurturer and homemaker:

> The industrial family ethic articulated the new arrangements of capitalism and patriarchy by linking the separation of the household and market work to a sexual division of labor—a specific set of recognizable and not altogether unfamiliar gender roles in which male "providers" worked for wages and female "homemakers" remained at home. . . . Pious, inferior, subordinate, and confined to the home as before, the new industrial family ethic elevated marriage, motherhood and the overseeing of family life to new ideological heights. (Abramovitz 1988, 111)

At the turn of the century, during industrialization, men traded self-directed work situations in home-based cottage industries and farms for supervised and subordinated wage work in the public marketplace. Women, who used to work side by side with their husbands in household-based industries, were then relegated to unpaid, if highly idealized, homemaking and child-care work and further subordinated roles in the family. Thus, male wage earners traded work-place autonomy for strengthened socially and economically supported domination over their households (Abramovitz 1988).

Currently, the ideological elevation of marriage and motherhood continues to buttress women's emotional commitment to unpaid mothering work. The price many American women pay for the performance of mothering work is some form of economic dependence on a male breadwinner or the invisible male provider, the state. The value of home-making and child rearing to the individual male breadwin-ner or the state is calculated neither as social value (power) in the gender relations within the patriarchal family nor as a component of the cost analysis of the necessary welfare services to legitimate state authority. Gillian Pascall (1986), a feminist state theorist, sums up the role of child care in women's dependency:

> The care of most dependents has been the province of women, has belonged to the domestic arena, and has been unpaid. It has thus made women dependent. . . . Feminist social policy, then, has been concerned with dependency, with the dependency of women, and of children, of elderly and handicapped people (the ma-jority of whom are also women). It has been concerned with just how tightly the knot has been tied between the dependency of the caring and the dependency of the cared for. (29–30)

Economic relations alone cannot explain the persistence of women's primary responsibility for home and child care. We also need to examine the processes inherent in market economies as they interact with patriarchy. It is important to uncover the assumptions about the family and the role of women implicit in current policies. Unpaid home and child-care work is essential to social policy, the sex-gender system of the division of labor, and the legitimation of the modern welfare state as the supposed provider of needed services. Current state policies that claim to support the family in fact support the breadwinner-dependent form of family, while explicitly penalizing alternate family forms (such as women-headed households) or families dependent on the state. Current social and economic arrangements require women's continuing emotional and ideological commitment to home and children. Despite the seemingly fragmentary nature of the provision of public services, there is a historical basis and an internal consistency to the tendency of social welfare policies to uphold women's unpaid caregiving roles (Pascall 1986, Quadagno 1987).

Individual women mother because, for many, becoming a mother also means becoming an adult. Performing mothering responsibilities adequately, particularly under the conditions in which many of our interviewees found themselves, is a tremendous challenge. Mothers who fail to meet this challenge experience terrible personal and social consequences.

On a macrolevel, what feminists refer to as the industrial family ethic has provided the political framework for the enduring idealization of motherhood. Women's primary responsibility for child care and homemaking is integral to the legitimation of the modern state as the supposed provider of needed services. The majority of our study participants depended on that invisible male provider, the social welfare service system, for support.

The Fiscal Crisis of the State

Economic growth in the United States after World War II created taxing and spending policies that afforded national financing of a wide array of services for problem populations. In this context, social welfare programs proliferated. In the 1970s, however, when this historic cycle of growth came to an end, what O'Connor (1973) has called "the fiscal crisis of the state" became a palpable reality. Simply put, the fiscal crisis was the growing excess of demand for services over the capacity for financing them.

Thus, in human services, there has been a trend in the 1980s and 1990s for social welfare programs to change from the federally mandated and funded programs developed in the 1960s to the state-by-state directed programs funded through federal block grant mechanisms promulgated during the Reagan and Bush administrations. As a result of shrinking state budgets, numerous social service programs have moved to public subsidization supervised by local governments and finally to privatization or the purchase of privately produced services. Historically, human service program provision tends to be downsized and funding increasingly privatized as programs move from federal to state to local supervision (Feldstein 1988).

For example, in March 1995 Congress debated the restructuring of the fifty-year-old federally mandated school lunch program. Republican proponents of the proposed legislation claimed that this restructuring was mandatory to address their campaign promises to balance the federal budget. Democratic adversaries responded that if school lunch programs were not protected at the federal level, individual states embroiled in their own political battles to balance budgets would downsize, defund, and eventually eliminate these essential services. Traditionally, federally mandated school lunch programs have ensured that approximately 3 million children in this country, whose families live below the poverty line, receive at least one nutritious meal per day. Such basic nutrition seems minimal while children learn the most basic skills necessary to function in society: reading, writing, and arithmetic.

Vincente Navarro (1986), a medical sociologist who analyzed trends in national and international health care provision, reminds us that such radical restructuring of the social welfare system "cannot take place only by repression but has to rely on active ideological offensive that could create a new consensus around a new set of values, beliefs and practices" (145). Employing Navarro's suggested analytical lens, we can examine how the media images of pregnant crack smokers as inhuman monsters during the late 1980s and early 1990s can be understood as such an active ideological offensive. We contend that the social construction of the so-called "crack baby" functioned to legitimate the downsizing and defunding of services for poor women and their children in the inner cities, who were also disproportionately women and children of color.

Beginning in 1988, a new social problem, crack, captured the nation's attention (Reinarman and Levine 1989, 1997). The image of poor inner-city African Americans, whose mothering instincts had been destroyed by crack, was highly publicized and widely accepted (Humphries 1999). Numerous media stories reported that the coming generation would comprise untold numbers of permanently impaired crack babies. Journalists predicted that these impaired infants would topple the health care delivery and educational systems due to their expensive and lifelong problems. At the same time, however, there was no comparable public discourse concerning the likelihood of huge expenditures of public resources for a much larger group of problematic infants, "tobacco babies," despite considerable available scientific evidence documenting the serious implications for the unborn of maternal tobacco smoking (Armstrong,

McDonald, and Sloan 1992; McDonald, Armstrong, and Sloan 1992).

In 1991, findings began to emerge contradicting previous predictions about pregnant crack users who were creating a "bio-underclass," or generation of permanently impaired children. It now appeared that the relationship between maternal crack smoking and fetal morbidity was far from clear (Chasnoff 1992, Coles et al. 1992, Lutiger et al. 1991). Poverty and lack of prenatal care were, in all probability, more significant contributing factors for the symptoms attributed to maternal crack smoking. Other important work was done on crack-exposed children indicating that, with proper care and parenting, by school age they developed on par with their unexposed peers (Barth 1991, Coles et al. 1992). During the same time, there was no political move to jail tobacco-smoking pregnant women, force them to go to treatment, or take away their children. Tobacco smoking was viewed as an unfortunate habit that pregnant women should try to avoid. By contrast, crack-smoking pregnant women and mothers were jailed or sentenced to treatment, or they lost custody of their children (Humphries et al. 1992, Humphries 1999, Siegel 1990). Clearly crack dealers did not have as much political power as the managers of the tobacco industry. As Joseph Gusfield's (1981) important work on the development of public problems indicates, the capacity of certain groups to never have their situations labeled "public problems" is a measure of their political power.

There are ideological explanations for why these infants continued to be labeled "crack babies" rather than, in light of scientific findings, "poverty babies." In an era of fiscal retrenchment, the notion of poverty babies might engender public sympathy and interfere with the conservative drive to demolish social welfare programs.

The discourse continued to be manipulated to construct public images of urban recipients of federal entitlement programs (such as Aid to Families with Dependent Children) as unfit mothers selling their children's food stamps to buy their next crack rock. Such images performed a legitimating function for legislators who were trying to promote social policies that would reduce resources for all poor women and children, whether or not they abused drugs (Maher 1992). The fiscal crisis of the state refers to the growing excess of demand for services without the required revenues for funding. Throughout the past two decades, the administration of human welfare programs has been turned over to state and local governments, which has usually resulted in shrinking service provision. This has coincided with an onslaught of negative media depictions of women on welfare, particularly women of color, as undeserving of public support due to their presumed drug abuse and child neglect.

The current policy context is one of fiscal retrenchment and diminished public support for social welfare services. Nonetheless, to begin to address the problems that our study participants experienced, federal funding for social welfare programs needs to be substantially increased, not cut.

Policy Implications

Policies that support families by providing guaranteed family income, housing, help with employment (when appropriate) and other sorts of ancillary services would have better served the women in our study when they were children. These policies would certainly have served them as mothers. The institution of a national health service, with women-oriented drug treatment, would ensure that all women and their children have access to comprehensive health care over their entire life.

Health and social welfare programs enabling families to stay together while a mother receives education, drug treatment, and help with parenting are the most promising roads back to conventional roles for mothers. Legislative, legal, and political practices that obstruct a mother's continuing contact or involvement with her children or send her to jail serve only to destroy the relationship critical to the stability and well-being of both the mother and child.

Child Removal

Beginning in the late 1980s, there has been a staggering increase in the number of children removed from their biological parents' custody:

Our survey of all fifty states' child welfare agencies revealed an unprecedented surge in the number of children removed from their parents and placed in foster care. APWA (American Public Welfare Association) estimates that, in June 1987, there were about 280,000 children in foster care; by June of 1990 the number is projected to increase to 360,000. That is a 29 percent increase in just 36 months—and the numbers are still rising. (Besharov 1990, 24)

California and New York together are responsible for 55 percent of the increase, and children of color have been grossly overrepresented. In 1990 in California, for the first time in the state's history, the absolute number of African-American children in foster care exceeded the number of whites, even though fewer than 10 percent of the state's children are African American (Besharov 1990, 25).

Child removal policies were also in vogue in the nineteenth century; then, like today, the children of the poor were overrepresented in institutions.

Distrust of the poor meant that children of poor, im-
migrant, and single mothers were over represented
among those removed from their families. Some mothers (and fathers) who could not care for their children
placed them in institutions voluntarily. Other children
were removed from their homes due to legitimate dis-
coveries of child abuse and neglect. But large numbers
of poor parents lost the right to raise their own children because they were seen as deviating from prescribed homemaker and breadwinner roles. (Abramovitz 1988, 167)

By the end of the nineteenth century, child removal policies lost their political support: "The earlier preference for
breaking up families as the most morally and economically
efficient method of enforcing prevailing work and family
norms and maintaining the future labor force lost some, if
not all, of its favor" (Abramovitz 1988, 170).

The twentieth-century rationale for child removal is also
based upon poor families' deviation from socially prescribed
drug-using patterns. Today, women who use illegal drugs
are at risk of having their children removed from their homes
and institutionalized or placed in foster care. In the early
years of this century, policies supporting placement of children in their own or foster care situations were instituted
and implemented. In the late 1980s and early 1990s, social
welfare practices returned to policies that prevailed in the
previous century.

As we should have learned from historical child removal
practices, children may not always be best served by removing them from their families. Foster care is often little better than the conditions from which children were removed.
It also lacks the caring of the natural mother, one of the few
sources of comfort for children in a frightening world.

The women we interviewed who lost custody of their children through CPS interventions were up against tremendous odds to regain custody. They needed to keep court dates and demonstrate proof of drug treatment, stable housing, and attendance at parenting classes. These hurdles were huge for single women lacking quality education, housing assistance, or welfare benefits and having minimal job experience or training. The few women who had job experience were more likely to be able to reenter the working world. Mothers whose families kept their children in informal arrangements had fewer obstacles to regaining custody.

As we have outlined, being a mother was the basis for most women's sense of self and social worth. When their children were forcibly removed, they lost the only shred of positive self-image left to them. There was no longer any reason not to be high all the time. The guilt, worry, and pain that these women experienced when their children were out of sight often provided another reason for continued heavy drug use and loss of control.

Housing

While many of their male partners bounced in and out of jail, many of our interviewees and children were "doing time" in SRO hotels and housing projects. In addition to the deplorable conditions of the majority of these dwellings, the prevalence of drug selling, using, and violence in these neighborhoods was staggering. Our interviewees described their housing projects as strewn with dead bodies, with children afraid to sit in front of windows for fear of being shot. Rhonda's description haunted the PAD staff:

Interviewer: Tell me some more about where you were living.
Rhonda: The way they [the housing projects] used to be they was tall buildings and short buildings, stone, concrete, a concrete jungle, babies would fall out

> the windows, babies would come out the house, be coming down the stairs underneath these little windows on the stairs, you would see babies falling from like eleven floors on down, falling out the windows, hitting on the pavement. People getting throwed out the windows, people coming in selling drugs, shooting drugs anywhere they please. Dead bodies here, dead bodies there.

When the women spoke longingly of living "anywhere but here," the appeal of what Waldorf (1973) called the geographic cure (moving away from the places in which one has used drugs) was understandable.

What might be the impact of constant, ambient violence on a developing fetus? While scant research has been conducted in the United States, we might begin to extrapolate (while keeping in mind the potential cultural differences) from a fascinating study conducted in Chile by Zapata and colleagues (1992) from the University of California at Berkeley. The goal of the study was to measure the impact on pregnancy outcomes of living in a highly violent environment. Employing a retrospective study design, the researchers were able to compare differences in pregnancy outcomes between women living under high levels of sociopolitical violence and women living under less violent conditions. Zapata and colleagues concluded: "After adjusting for potential confounders, [we determined] that high levels of sociopolitical violence were associated with an approximately fivefold increase in risk of pregnancy complications" (1992, 689).

Housing projects held other hazards for women's and children's health (Bowman and Rojas 1995, Johnson 1994). For example, a news story during the summer of 1994 reported tenant complaints about conditions at Geneva Towers, a San Francisco public housing project. Many occupants complained of chronic exhaustion, severe headaches, hair loss, and runny eyes. The children who lived in the project were vomiting regularly and had persistent rashes over their bodies. All of the tenants contended that the source of their troubles was the rundown federally subsidized building in which they all lived.

A group of these tenants staged a protest at a board of supervisors meeting at city hall. They brought bottles full of foul-smelling brown water they had drawn from their kitchen taps. Although the Department of Public Health insisted that tests conducted six months previously showed that the water was fine, the tenants vehemently disagreed. The Department of Housing and Urban Development admitted that the water was sometimes rusty but insisted that it was not a health risk. Tenants, however, argued angrily that frequently their water smelled like human excrement.

The air was also a source for complaints since the ventilation system had been shut down for some time. One member of San Francisco's board of supervisors stated: "There have been a number of improvements over the last year or so at Geneva Towers, but it's still a pit. I wouldn't want to live there, and I don't think you would either" (Johnson 1994, A21).

These hazardous and dangerous living conditions were particularly ironic when one considers the long waiting lists to move into these housing projects. In May 1993, we interviewed a CPS worker about her work responsibilities. While enumerating the frustrations of her job, the social worker discussed the lengthy public housing waiting list:

It's the biggest issue. You can't find it. I mean, it's not available out there for you, and if I wanted to move, never mind someone who does not, you know, have a regular job and is on GA [General Assistance or Social

Security Income]. The availability is just pretty bad. I know someone who just got Section Eight housing, but she had her name on the list in '85.

Her client waited eight years to move into hazardous and perilous housing. To intervene effectively in poor women's and their children's lives, municipalities must provide available, safe, and affordable housing.

Guaranteed Family Income

If stable living environments for growing children are indeed a policy goal, then a guaranteed subsistence income for children and their caregivers would be cost-effective from both a fiscal and a humanistic perspective. For example, in New York City foster care payments for children less than five years old are two and one-half times higher than Aid to Families with Dependent Children (AFDC) payments for the same child (Besharov 1990). This figure begs the question, Why not raise payments on AFDC and ease the economic devastation that assuredly contributes to women's drug abuse? Why continue to pay more to nonbiological care givers than to birth parents?

Health Care

We believe that adequate health care should be available for all Americans. Other than South Africa, the United States is the only Western democracy that does not have some form of national health service. We do not believe that the United States is in very good company regarding its health care provision system.

That said, we now focus specifically on the provision of prenatal and reproductive health care for pregnant drug users. As we have detailed, what emerged from women's narratives was the irony of prenatal care as a risk factor rather than a risk-reduction strategy. Although some of the study participants had positive experiences, for many, seeking prenatal care was a source of anxiety and a maternal risk factor in and of itself.

Poland and colleagues (1993) interviewed 142 low-income postpartum women to determine their attitudes regarding possible effects of a punitive law on the behavior of substance-using pregnant women. The purpose of the study was to investigate women's attitudes about whether or not pregnant drug users should be prosecuted and to determine whether punitive legislation directed at this group would deter women from seeking prenatal care and participating in drug-treatment programs. The study's key finding was that the interviewees believed strongly that punitive legislation would further alienate pregnant drug users from seeking needed health care. These women were convinced that women would "go underground" to avoid detection and treatment for fear of incarceration and loss of custody of their children. This opinion was held both by women who did and did not use drugs during pregnancy. Several women interviewed noted that "these laws are just for poor black women, not rich white ones!" (Poland et al. 1993, 202).

Similarly, Chavkin, Allen, and Oberman (1991) suggest: "Attempts to criminalize drug use during pregnancy may further deter [pregnant women] from seeking care or from giving accurate information to health care providers. Anecdotal reports suggest that efforts to detect maternal drug use by means of urine toxicology testing of the newborn may even frighten some women away from delivering in hospitals" (107). Citing an article in the *Reproductive Rights Update*, Chavkin and colleagues (1991) go on to say that within the medical community sources note that in South Carolina, where prosecutors have filed criminal charges against women who allegedly used drugs during pregnancy, there has been a rise in the number of women giving birth at home, in taxis, and in bathrooms.

Clearly, punitive policies are counterproductive. While the connection between drug use and fetal impairment is ambiguous (with the notable exception of tobacco and alcohol), we do know that poor health in general, malnourishment, chronic stress, and illness certainly influence both mother and infant adversely. Our findings indicate that it is more beneficial to promote women's perceptions of health care as a part of the harm-reduction strategies they employ than to let health care constitute yet another risk in their lives.

Drug Treatment

Women's access to drug treatment has always been problematic due primarily to differential perceptions of gender-role obligations. Most inpatient drug-treatment programs do not accept children and are therefore incompatible with women's needs. A majority of inpatient treatment programs require a minimum thirty-day commitment, and some are as long as one year. For a woman with young children to care for, this can be an insurmountable obstacle (Daghestani 1988, Jessup and Green 1987).

In 1981, we commented on the findings from our qualitative study of one hundred women heroin addicts: "For a woman addict, live-in treatment is only possible when she has no other family commitments. For the 70 percent of the women in our sample who were mothers, treatment facilities without accommodations for children are worthless" (Rosenbaum and Murphy 1981, 4). Little has changed in the ensuing seventeen years. Women with substance-abuse problems are still unable, for the most part, to find inpatient services that will accommodate their children.

Those women who need outpatient services are also in

need of assistance with their child-care responsibilities. Programs that provide supervised play areas for children while their mothers receive counseling or medication are few and far between. Children are left to fend for themselves or are made privy to the content of counseling sessions for lack of any alternative (Reed 1987). Many women expressed fears of being found out—having their drug abuse discovered by their children. Treatment programs need to be sensitive to these maternal privacy needs (Finkelstein 1994, Mondanaro 1988, Murphy and Rosenbaum 1987, Reed 1987, Rosenbaum 1981).

A woman-sensitive approach to treatment is necessary to meet the multiple needs of this population. The main thrust of women-sensitive services is in planning and implementing programs designed specifically for women rather than asking women to conform to a male standard of care. A complete array of services not only takes into account recovery strategies tailored to women's needs but includes a number of ancillary services that allow women clients to derive the full benefit of available options. These ancillary services may include transportation, child care, children's health services, housing, legal assistance, and job or vocational training.

An important part of a woman's recovery from chemical dependency is the counseling aspect of a program. Counseling may take a variety of forms, depending upon the focus of the program. Group sessions may be offered by a program, including twelve-step programs such as Alcoholics Anonymous or Narcotics Anonymous. Individual counseling sessions with a psychotherapist or substance-abuse counselor may also be an important program attribute.

Additionally, family therapy is a crucial component of comprehensive drug treatment. Family therapy helps examine the family system as a unit and includes partners and others in the woman's treatment and recovery process. The few studies that have focused on treatment outcomes for women generally endorse a group format over individual therapy, family therapy as the most effective modality, separate treatment for men and women clients, and female therapists rather than male therapists (Baldwin et al. 1995, Gerskin and Harwood 1990).

Current treatment models for drug dependent women are based on male-oriented approaches. Whether this is due to the lack of available research or the smaller numbers of women in some kinds of treatment programs remains to be seen. It is known, however, that treatment programs are inadequate for women's needs and are not prepared to deal with the multiple needs of the chemically dependent pregnant woman (Baldwin et al. 1995; Cuskey, Berger, and Densen-Gerber 1977; Levy and Doyle 1974; Michaels et al. 1988; Mondanaro et al. 1982; Murphy and Rosenbaum 1987; Reed 1987; Reed et al. 1980; Rosenbaum 1981; Rosenbaum and Murphy 1987; Sterk 1998).

Viable Alternatives: Women-Sensitive Treatment

Inpatient programs that accept children, expansion (and, in some areas of the country, creation) of chemically dependent pregnancy clinics, special job training programs for women, and long-term commitment of funding for aftercare are some viable alternatives to present-day service modalities.

Women Only

The institution of women-only treatment programs would help to create a safe, nonexploitative environment in which women could recover. Male orientation and inherent sexism in treatment make some programs unsuitable for the woman in recovery (Levy and Doyle 1974; Soler, Onsor, and Abod 1976; Reed 1987). If separate programs are not feasible, the institution of women-only support groups would be satisfactory.

Pregnancy and Parenting

In 1990, Wendy Chavkin conducted a survey of drug treatment facilities throughout New York City. Her survey yielded the following findings:

> The general shortage of treatment slots is aggravated by the unwillingness of many drug programs to include pregnant women. A recent survey in New York by the author revealed that 54 percent of treatment programs categorically excluded the pregnant. Effective availability was further limited by restrictions on method of payment or specific substance of abuse. Sixty-seven percent of the programs rejected pregnant Medicaid patients and only 13 percent accepted pregnant Medicaid patients addicted to crack. (1990, 485)

Another survey conducted in the same year found that, of the approximately 675,000 pregnant women in need of drug treatment nationwide, fewer than 11 percent received it (Paltrow 1992). Most treatment facilities are unprepared and inadequate for the multiple needs of pregnant and chemically dependent women. Separate clinics or clinics within clinics must be institutionalized.

Treatment must deal with women's needs for parenting support. Facilities should provide parenting-skills training, referrals to appropriate agencies, and emergency help for mother and child survival needs. Regarding the effects of children on mothers' mental health, Shapiro, Perry, and Brewin (1979) report that no other factor relates as heavily to conflict as young children in the home. Inpatient programs that accept a woman and her children are absolutely necessary. Often, for the alcohol- or drug-misusing mother, strengthening her ability to parent may be the first important step in her eventual recovery. Drug-treatment programs must include support for women's roles as parents as well as meet child care needs as a central part of the treatment process (Messer, Anderson, and Martin 1996; Michaels et al. 1988; Rosenbaum and Murphy 1987).

Job Training and Aftercare

Women drug misusers (as well as men) need job training programs. If women do not have the ability to make a living, post-treatment reentry into conventional life will undoubtedly mean relapse into previous drug-abuse patterns. Aftercare (follow-up support and counseling when program has been completed) demands long-term funding commitments to both evaluate programs and support successful reentry. Facilitating creation of women-sensitive drug-treatment services will require the participation of treatment consumers, providers, and policymakers.

In order for women-sensitive treatment to develop, clients need to be supported in the formulation of advocacy-style self-help groups so that they can influence the formulation of treatment policy. Such organizations would go a long way toward combating the depression, isolation, and low self-esteem that persists among women in treatment (Beckman 1978; Messer, Anderson, and Martin 1996; Michaels et al. 1988; Mondanaro 1988; Murphy and Rosenbaum 1987; Reed 1987).

Treatment providers need to support client activism. Providers themselves require the sustenance that ongoing gender-specific training and frequent staff inservices furnish. Such training helps forestall burnout and increases program efficacy. Efforts must be made to undermine the forces of sexism, racism, elitism, and professionalism that divide health workers from one another and prevent them from realizing common interests (Waitzkin 1989). In a very real sense, drug-treatment health workers, like their clients, must mobilize against the negative forces of degradation and burnout that come with this occupation (Zweben and Sorensen 1988). Finally, both staff and clients must educate public policymakers (such as legislators) about the ever-changing needs of this treatment population.

The Political Economy of Drug Treatment

Estes and colleagues (1984), in their discussion of the commodification of health and the aging enterprise, assert:

> What is most relevant to our concern with health and aging is that business and government have begun to look at medical care as more nearly an economic product than a social good. Within this context, the incentive is to maximize profits rather than health. The consequence for the elderly, for all persons dependent on public policy and programs, is that social needs are turned into profit-making commodities. (1984, 19)

The commodification of drug-abuse treatment must be avoided. Drug abusers, especially women with substance-abuse problems, are extremely vulnerable players in the public policy arena. The disastrous consequences of leaving this population untreated, due to the development of a drug industry enterprise without publicly funded alternatives, will be with us for generations to come.

The United States claims to be in the midst of waging a war on drugs. The battle is being fought with meager weapons when it comes to the treatment of substance-abusing women. Women who seek help with their abuse problems face adversity in three areas: access, cost, and quality. The most significant barrier to access is the lack of facilities for children. Drug and alcohol programs are prohibitively expensive for women. Programs for women are often exploitative, sexist, and, in the main, oriented toward male clients.

Facilitating the creation of women-sensitive treatment services will require the participation of treatment consumers, providers, and policymakers. These three groups must be mobilized to prevent the creation of a drug-treatment enterprise without publicly funded alternatives, leaving women and children without necessary services.

Many women in our study population had been used and abused since birth, with adult relatives and guardians sexually assaulting or emotionally abusing them throughout their childhoods. If they were placed in foster care, that system often failed to protect them as well. Home problems interfered with schooling, and lack of quality education decreased job opportunities. Teenage pregnancies truncated childhoods. Many of the interviewees were babies who had babies. Violence was everywhere—in their own homes, in the next project apartment, and outside on the streets. The 1990s brought a different and, in some ways, more virulent kind of abuse. Pregnant drug users were now used as part of a larger ideological offensive to legitimate the wholesale reduction of social welfare services to all poor women and children. We believe that history may prove this last to be the most devastating abuse of all.

Women's drug use during pregnancy reveals more about the low point in social conditions in American cities than about the powers of any particular drug. Our unrealistic social expectations for women, discrimination in hiring, and the lack of a national health care system and social services for women and children all conspire to block legitimate routes to satisfaction and well-being. Women's drug use during pregnancy cannot be understood apart from the social and economic contexts in which these experiences were embedded. The greatest threat to effective parenting and child survival is a system that perpetuates poverty, violence, hardship, and desperation. Rather than indicting pregnant drug users for their addictions and compulsions, we would do well to look at the impossible conditions in which these women and their children are forced to live their lives.

Appendix 1

Women Talking to Women: Methodological and Theoretical Perspectives

We chose an exploratory study design to gather information from the women's own perspectives and in their own voices. We embraced a theoretical perspective appropriate for exploration: (1) the philosophy of phenomenology that places the view of the actor and her meaning-making process at the center of analysis and (2) symbolic interactionism that stresses the importance of meaning, language, and interaction (Becker 1970, Blumer 1969, Charon 1995, Geertz 1973, Mead 1939, Schutz 1967, Spradley 1979). We relied on concepts such as social role, identity, process, and, most of all, understanding life as our participants saw it. In this effort, we appreciated the timeless words of John Lofland (1971):

> The commitment to get close, to be factual, and descriptive and quotive, constitutes a significant commitment to represent the participants in their own terms. This does not mean that one becomes an apologist for them, but rather that one faithfully depicts what goes on in their lives and what life is like for them, in such a way that one's audience is at least partially able to project themselves into the point of view of the people depicted. They can "take the role of the other" because the reporter has given them a living sense of day-to-day talk, and day-to-day activities, day-to-day concerns and problems. The audience can know the

petty vexations of their existence, the disappointments that befall them, the joys and triumphs they savor, the typical contingencies they face. There is a conveyance of their prides, their shames, their secrets, their fellowships, their boredoms, their happinesses, their despairs.

A major methodological consequence of this commitment is that the qualitative study of people *in situ* is a process of discovery. One must find out what the subjects themselves believe they are doing in their own terms rather than impose a preconceived or outsider's scheme of what they are doing. (4)

Both of the authors are medical sociologists trained at the University of California, San Francisco, and a cornerstone of our theoretical training was phenomenology and symbolic interactionism. We are also influenced by the newer postmodern/feminist perspectives. Laurel Richardson's (1994) explication of the core of postmodernism summarizes this world view:

The core of postmodernism is the *doubt* that any method or theory, discourse or genre, tradition or novelty, has a universal and general claim as the "right" or the privileged form of authoritative knowledge. Postmodernism *suspects* all truth claims of masking and serving particular interests in local, cultural, and political struggles. But postmodernism does not automatically reject conventional methods of knowing and telling as false or archaic. Rather, it opens those standard methods to inquiry and introduces new methods, which are also, then, subject to critique. (518)

Through postmodernism, we were sensitized by

Criticisms of empirical qualitative work, such as bias, questions about adequacy or credibility, relationships with persons in the research, and ethical implications . . . whose voices are heard and how, and whether text or experience should be created, and by whom. (Olesen 1994, 167)

Although seasoned researchers, we had to incorporate into our research process the postmodern critique of previous qualitative work. We planned the pregnancy and drug-use study with these methodological challenges in mind. We were no longer unabashedly seeking "truth" because postmodern thought had deconstructed the idea of scientific validity and replaced it with interpretation (Denzin 1994). To honor the politics of interpretation by displaying our interpretive process, (1) the language text had to be preserved, and (2) the voice of both the subject and researcher had to be acknowledged.

In previous writings, we attempted to present participants' world views and saw ourselves as intellectual descendants of a long line of sympathetic spokeswomen for the underdog (Becker 1963, Irwin 1970, Matza 1969). With the postmodern influence on qualitative methods, it became even more important to let the words and experiences of interviewees speak for themselves while recognizing our own standpoints, perspectives, and limitations. Thus, who *we* are is extremely relevant for our readers' evaluations of the resulting interpretations. The reader, therefore, will find us woven throughout this report, sometimes in the first person singular, sometimes in the first person plural. Six of us worked on this project at different stages. As our friend Professor Troy Duster reminds us, "Scratch an ideology and you come up with a biography."

Feminist theory provided the study's methodological link among phenomenology, symbolic interactionism, and postmodernism. The most pronounced value of feminist methods, we believe, is the explicit introduction of humanity into research (Olesen 1994). Although attention to the postmodern critique influenced the formulation of the study, principles of feminist research strongly influenced how we envisioned our research process. Since the study population comprised only pregnant women, feminist methods provided a more humane, interactive, and equitable approach. Feminist methods require reflexivity among the researchers, sensitivity to the interviewer-interviewee relationship, and the input of study participants in both data collection and analysis.

Grounded theory proved most useful and effective for an interactive process of data collection and analysis. This method is based on the notion that data should be collected and analyzed in a way that allows the basic social, social-psychological, and structural processes inherent in any phenomenon to emerge naturally (Glaser and Strauss 1970; Glaser 1978; Strauss 1987; Strauss and Corbin 1990, 1994). We tried (not always successfully) to clear our minds of preconceived ideas about the experience of pregnancy and drug use and to listen to what the women told us about their lives. Each interview added new information and posed new questions, and the grounded theory method of combining data collection and analysis was most compatible with our study's focus.

We were students of varied disciplines and modes of scientific inquiry, but we all shared a feminist perspective. Marsha Rosenbaum is a product of the blurred genres and early feminism of 1970–86; Sheigla Murphy and Katherine Irwin were students of later, more developed feminisms and the crisis of representation from 1986 to the present (Denzin and Lincoln 1994, Krieger 1991, Van Maanen 1988). Margaret Kearney was a doctoral candidate in nursing, Kim Theidon in anthropology; and Jeanette Irwin was in an international relations graduate program. Murphy, Rosenbaum, and Kearney were mothers in their late thirties and early forties, and only Rosenbaum was married. Theidon and the Irwin sisters were younger women in their early to late twenties, and they more closely mirrored the ages of our study participants. Although our ethnicities varied (Jewish, Irish, Italian, German), we shared with each other the triple statuses of race (Caucasian), class (middle), and education (postgraduate degrees).

We wanted to create an interview context in which our study participants felt that their perspectives were privileged and their stories would be heard. The interviewees were to be the experts on the phenomena of interest—pregnancy and drug use. A reflexive methodology that allowed the interviewees to decide what the important interview topics would be was absolutely necessary. Qualitative, grounded theory methods were appropriate and most effective at achieving these goals.

We unabashedly wanted to influence policy in favor of pregnant drug users, to contribute to turning the tide of intolerance, to facilitate positive change for these women who had been so quickly and unfairly judged in ways that smacked more than a little of racism and elitism. Our method also had to reflect our status as drug-abuse experts committed to rigorous scientific inquiry in order to open dialogue with policymakers. We employed feminist qualitative methods to remove the hyphen between the researcher and the researched (Fine 1994), and at the same time we attended to the study's scientific rigor so that those in power might listen to our recommendations.

Data Collection

Inclusion Criteria

The study population consisted of 120 adult (age eighteen or older) women in the San Francisco Bay Area who were pregnant or no more than six months' postpartum. Interviewees must have used either heroin, cocaine, or methamphetamine (or any combination thereof) for a minimum of twenty-five days during their current or most recent pregnancy. Women who were enrolled in drug treatment for more than five days within a five-week period were not included in the study. Those women who were in treatment for less than five days had to have returned to drug use for five or more days since their last day of treatment. These criteria allowed us to interview women who had had brief encounters with drug treatment and had since reestablished their drug-use patterns. Thus, we were able to explore reasons for leaving treatment.

Based on our past research and the relevant literature, we divided pregnancy into three stages. Stage 1 women were between two and twenty weeks' pregnant.[1] Stage 2 women were between twenty-one weeks' pregnant to delivery or termination. Stage 3 participants could be no more than six months' postpartum.[2]

To fully explore AIDS risks, attitudes, and behaviors, we made sure that half (twenty) of the women interviewed in each stage were intravenous drug users (IDUs). IDUs were defined as those women who had injected heroin, cocaine, or methamphetamine at least once a week during the six months before discovering their pregnancy. These inclusion criteria allowed us to examine the changes in drug administration before and after the onset of pregnancy. A noninjection drug user was defined as any woman who had not injected drugs in the previous two years. Each subgroup, IDU and non-IDU, in each of the three stages of pregnancy contained twenty subjects. Our past research had demonstrated that a minimum of twenty interviews was necessary to discover meaningful patterns and produce a robust theoretical framework.

Sampling Strategy and Recruitment

We used a modified version of Watters and Biernacki's (1989) targeted sampling to recruit our study population. This combined theoretical sampling (Strauss 1987), quota sampling (Kalton 1983), and chain-referral sampling (Biernacki and Waldorf 1981). The combination of methods was particularly well suited to our study because it allowed us to locate and recruit subjects. At the same time, we circumvented limitations associated with convenience sampling, such as nonrepresentativeness and the systematic exclusion of interviewees in harder-to-recruit racial and social class groups (Babbie 1986). While targeted samples are not random samples, they are also not convenience samples. Rather, they entail a strategy to obtain systematic data when true random sampling is not feasible and when convenience sampling is not rigorous enough to meet the assumptions of the research design (Watters and Biernacki 1989).

Initially, we developed race and social class quotas for each of the three stages of pregnancy. Although the demographic characteristics of the population studied had not been extensively documented, there was sufficient available information on race and social class to support the development of quotas (Chasnoff, Landress, and Barrett 1990; Skolnick 1990).

Once quotas had been developed, we used a chain-referral method to locate our participants. This method had been used regularly by sociologists, ethnographers, and social psychologists working in deviant, illegal, sensitive, or private subject areas (Biernacki and Waldorf 1981, McBride and Clayton 1985). Several authors of classic drug studies used chain-referral recruitment, among them Becker (1963), Feldman (1968), Lindesmith (1968), Preble and Casey (1969), and Waldorf (1973).

More recently, this method has been employed to locate hard-to-find groups such as women heroin addicts (Rosenbaum 1981), needle sharers (Murphy 1987), untreated heroin addicts (Waldorf and Biernacki 1981), crack-using women (Murphy forthcoming), and cocaine users and quitters (Waldorf, Reinarman, and Murphy 1991). Contacts from past projects helped us to find locators, who then acted as recruiters. These individuals were current and ex-users who were informed of study inclusion criteria and were paid a locator fee of twenty dollars for every completed interview.

The chain-referral method worked as follows: one interviewee referred us to friends within her social scene. The referred interviewee then referred us to others within her social world or to potential interviewees within different but related scenes, thus forming chains of participants. Project staff kept close track of the ethnic and social-class memberships in each of our three stages. They stopped interviewing when quotas were met or began new chains in new drug-using groups when necessary.

We recruited interviewees by publicizing our study in public areas. We posted colorful flyers describing our study in food distribution centers, laundromats, bars, restaurants, and coffee houses and on telephone poles all over the city. We tried to post fliers in hospital and clinic waiting rooms. That was often difficult since most of the health care and social service providers were reticent about cooperating in order to protect their clients. Gatekeepers at private facilities serving middle-class women were especially protective and refused to allow us to post informational signs in their waiting rooms. Our most successful recruitment method was the chain-referral method. We believe that the stigma conferred on pregnant drug users discouraged many women from participating in the project. We speculate that the forty-dollar honorarium provided incentive for impoverished users and that middle-class women with more resources were not willing to reveal their drug use even with the promise of confidentiality. As a result, despite our considerable effort to recruit middle-class women, the majority of our sample lived at or beneath the poverty line.

The Qualitative Interview Guide

Although we had some specific research questions, the study was primarily exploratory. Our goal was to provide a thick description of salient aspects of drug use in pregnancy. Since little was known about this population, we used a semi-structured interview guide. The guide contained broad topical areas to be covered but did not limit responses to predetermined, or close-ended, responses. Open-ended questions were necessary to get a description of a woman's situation and social world and to capture her experience and the meaning she attached to it.

Our interview took the form of a life history and covered the individual's "story" from birth to the present. We solicited details about the women's drug use, particularly while pregnant. We had the advantage of having consistent topic areas related to our research questions while allowing new topic areas to emerge. Our research began with a set of sensitizing concepts. These were preliminary notions about the categories, relationships, and problems we had found during our previous research. The interview began with a family history, an education profile, and work (including illegal jobs) and relationship history. Interview questions explored the introduction and initiation to drug use, the social environments of use, pressures to use or not use, and the relationship of pregnancy to patterns of drug use. Types of drugs used, amounts used, frequency of use, and combinations of drugs used were discussed as well as modes of administration, including injecting, smoking, and internasal use. In sum, the qualitative interview guide was designed to tap the entire experience of the pregnant drug user in order to elicit a thick description.

Quantitative Measures

Our structured instrument enabled us to collect relevant demographic data as well as drug-use history and patterns. Additionally, we included measures of needle sharing and high-risk AIDS sexual practices. The quantitative interview schedule consisted of a set of short-answer and precoded questions pertaining to basic life history information and patterns of drug use during pregnancy. Questions were designed to collect information regarding family of origin, work and education, arrests and criminal activities, violence, frequency of use, methods of drug administration, family and marital relations, and chronological history of drug use with an emphasis on the current pregnancy.

The Depth Interview

Locations. We conducted interviews in a variety of settings: residence hotels, where we sometimes had to pay five dollars and leave an ID at the door to visit an interviewee; treatment facilities; participants' homes, and (as a last resort) our offices. We wanted to interview women in the setting in which they would be most comfortable and feel free to speak candidly. This required privacy, but many women did not have the kind of living arrangement in which two to four hours of private time was possible.

Establishing Trust. The purpose of scientific study instruments is to collect valid and reliable data. Traditionally, social scientists have aspired, in this way, to get the truth from their subjects. In an attempt to do real science, however, so-called rigorous methodologies are often at odds with the collection of valid and meaningful data. Study participants are literally subjected to a barrage of questions, many of them difficult or annoying to answer. Often interviewees have no motivation to tell the truth or elaborate. They simply want to collect the honorarium and leave.

Our first priority was to elicit information so that we could fully understand pregnancy and drug use. We were concerned that our procedures might offend study participants and exacerbate feelings of shame that would make them leery of us from the beginning. It was essential that subjects trust us in order to feel comfortable divulging sensitive personal information (that theoretically could be used against them in custody disputes, for example) about their complex, often criminal, and nearly always problematic lives. We had to trust that their accounts, which were our sole source of information, were truthful because we had no way of substantiating their stories without betraying confidentiality.

Establishing Rapport. Participants' trust that we would not disclose any information was very precarious and only achieved after some time of getting acquainted and establishing rapport. Since this one aspect of the research process was absolutely essential to the collection of meaningful data, we had to structure our interview process to achieve that rapport.

Consistent with feminist goals of mutuality and relationality (Hall and Stevens 1991), we tried to anticipate women's special needs. To begin, once the pre-interview procedures had been completed, we offered food and drink. If we were in their home, we behaved like invited guests, accepting their offerings. We worked at establishing rapport by demonstrating respect and relying on gender as a common ground.

Fontana and Frey (1994) have considered the issue of respect:

> There is growing reluctance, especially among female researchers (Oakley 1981; Reinharz 1992; Smith 1987) to continue interviewing women as "objects," with little or no regard for them as individuals. Whereas this reluctance stems from moral and ethical issues, it is also very relevant methodologically. . . . Thus the emphasis is shifting to allow the development of a closer relation between interviewer and respondent, attempting to minimize status differences and doing away with the traditional hierarchical situation in interviewing. (370)

The pregnant women we interviewed were doubly stigmatized and therefore treated with little respect, not only in conventional settings but within their own social worlds. Most had no safe place to talk about using drugs while pregnant. We told them that we were interested in *their* story, that their story would be compared with other women's experiences to generate common themes. We stressed that they, not we, were the experts in this prolonged conversation. In this effort, we used a conversational style, described by Field and colleagues (1994) in this way:

> The deliberate choice of conversation as a process of data collection assumes an attitude toward the research

and the participants that is significant and different from the technique of interview. This difference may be that of a dependence on *tact* in creating the conversation, as opposed to a reliance on the preconceived *tactic* of a structured questionnaire. (9)

We believe that this conversational style made the interview feel safer, less like an interrogation and more like two women getting to know one another. Some women were embarrassed, saying they had not talked this much about themselves in a long time. As we relied on them to make sense of their worlds, they sharpened our analysis, essentially helping us by doing our work for us.

We placed the interviewees at center stage, encouraging them to tell their story from their perspective. We emphasized from the outset there were no right or wrong answers possible. Instead, the woman became the center of the process, and we became the facilitators of the conversation. If they chose to expound on a subject, that was all right. If not, we did not push for elaboration because we wanted them to continue to feel comfortable.

Pregnant addicts are constantly dealing with individuals who want them to change. We appreciated them as they were and made it clear that we were interested in research, not social work or therapy. Some women wanted advice or information, and we referred them to appropriate agencies or programs. We were interested in their lives and their strategies for negotiating their worlds rather than who was to blame for their problems and what they should be doing.

We were six white middle-class women who were interviewing mostly underclass women from diverse races and ethnicities. Thus, we did not share class or race membership. Ultimately, the common ground was gender. Very quickly we made contact on the most obvious and perhaps the only basis possible—as women. Through joking or just acknowledgment (about men, children, or other problems that women share), a connection was made between two people who came from very different social worlds but shared gendered life experiences.

For a few hours, we got to know each other, talking with

the women about men, sex, pregnancy, the difficulties of being a single mother, money, and child-care issues. For those of us who were mothers, our roles as mothers helped in immeasurable ways. We understood maternal feelings: their struggles to keep their children and raise them properly; their pain and frustration when, as often happened, things did not go as they hoped and planned.

We laughed often about children and at the expense of men. We joked about how hard it was to have kids, how they could drive you crazy, how difficult it is to be a mother. Most of our interviewees were single parents, and so were a couple of our interviewers. All the interviewers shared relationship problems. We laughed (and sometimes cried) about the problems of living with and without men. The transcripts were indicative of the interactive and not merely question-and-answer nature of the interviews. A passage in which the interviewee discussed problems she'd had with an unsupportive male was often followed by another long passage by an interviewer who could identify with her situation. Our study participants, while anxious to return to their own story, appreciated our support.

The key to establishing rapport with our study participants was that we were women interviewing other women. This has everything to do with socialization into traditional gender roles (Chodorow 1978). Such roles emphasize listening skills: understanding and making central the perspectives and needs of others. Women learn to analyze and find solutions to others' problems; they realize that survival as a female depends on taking the role of the other. Each of these characteristics makes for an extremely skilled interviewer, and we believe they are imperative for interviewing women.

Traditionally, women have less difficulty than men asking for help, advice, and information. Some of the women on our staff were young; relatively inexperienced with research; and apparently naïve, vulnerable, and harmless (Warren 1988). Many interviewees felt that it was appropriate to adopt these well-meaning but naïve researchers, offering to school them in the ways of the drug life.

Seventy percent of the participants had been victims of violence by the men in their lives. As a consequence, they were less trusting of men than of women and more likely to feel comfortable with a woman interviewer. Nevertheless, even though we were able to establish reasonable rapport most of the time, interviewer and interviewee did not always click. Fortunately, this was a rare occurrence. Even if a few women were reticent to talk, there was always something to be learned from every interview encounter.

Researchers can encounter any number of problems with rapport: "going native," speaking for the group being studied, and losing objectivity (Fontana and Frey 1994), all of which can blur the delicate line between researcher and researched. Nobody on the staff became pregnant (although we did joke about it all the time), nor do we even pretend to be able to speak for pregnant drug users. We were able, however, to establish rapport with the women in our study population most of the time.

Pregnant and postpartum addicts constantly lived with the threat of losing custody of their children to CPS. Although they often asked for assistance, it was frustrating for us to be for the most part unable to help them with this problem. One woman told us about the day her children were taken away. They were screaming and their faces were pressed up against the windows of the CPS bus. These children loved their mother, and she loved them. She chased the bus for blocks. Following their removal from her home, she went on a crack binge. She tried to get them back and often visited the home where one of the foster parents was abusing her son. At the end of the interview, she asked for our help in getting her children back, but we could do nothing but refer her to an agency that helped reunify families.

We heard about terrible violence from the women we interviewed. Many lived with men who routinely beat them while they were pregnant. They were often hit or kicked in the stomach. Their children were abused. Still, we could do nothing unless they asked for a referral.

As intravenous users of drugs or those engaging in unsafe sex, many of the women and their children were at risk for contracting HIV. One of the most heart-wrenching accounts came from a woman who was HIV positive. She delivered her baby alone, and, discovering that it was stillborn, put it into the garbage. The staff member who conducted the interview wrote in her field notes:

> That was hard. She told me the whole story about that. And what was even harder about it was that she would address me by name during the interview. She would constantly engage me in her story by saying my name. It was especially difficult because it was really a bonding feeling. It usually feels really nice when someone addresses you by name because they are paying attention to you. It's not just that they're on stage, but they're giving you something and they are including you in the story. But this was not a story in which anyone would feel comfortable being included. She was pregnant and she was kicked out of her house and she went on a crack binge and she moved into a motel and she was tossing up and she went into labor and she gave birth to a child and it was dead and she cut the umbilical cord and put it [the baby] in the garbage.

We especially felt the frustration, after establishing rapport and including the women in the research process, of knowing that this interview might be the only bright spot in their lives for a very long time. Regardless of their motivations for change and temporary achievements, most were likely, lacking other options, to return eventually to a drug-, violence-, and risk-inundated life. Not only did we feel unhelpful in concrete ways, but we knew, sadly, that the women's own best efforts were a long shot at best, given their socioeconomic and stigmatized statuses.

Despite our rapport-creating efforts through shared gendered experiences and a conversational style of interviewing, we remained white middle-class women interviewing for the most part underclass women of color. These differences, we believe, perpetuated at least some degree of mistrust. We were, after all, professionals and "white folks," like the social workers, hospital personnel, and others who had influenced interviewees' lives in a mostly negative way. True mutuality was impossible.

Qualitative Data Analysis

Immediately following the interview, we generated key descriptive and narrative material. Also following the interview, we recorded our impressions and wrote a descriptive and analytic summary statement. The data were coded immediately after collection. It was imperative that as little time as possible elapse between collection and initial analysis. While coding, we noted patterns that seemed potentially salient or recurrent. Through coding the data for salient dimensions, we discovered constellations of basic social, social-psychological, and structural processes. While coding the data, and certainly afterward, we wrote increasingly refined theoretical memos or scanned the data (Goetz and LeCompte 1984). This was the think work of the analysis. By making these memos, we began to conceptually connect the diverse codes and discern emerging patterns. Saturation was reached when there was continuing redundancy in memos about basic social processes and their properties across a number of diverse groups.

The analysis of our data occurred simultaneously with their collection. We studied the completed interviews for the purpose of alerting ourselves to those subject areas that stood out. In this way, we began to recognize the aspects of women's drug use during pregnancy that appeared most prominent. This enabled us to explore these areas further in subsequent interviews.

Coding

We coded the interview on the computer as soon as it was transcribed, using the qualitative management program known as *Ethnograph* (1989). The codes were derived directly from the interview transcripts and were subject areas that, by virtue of the time the interviewee spent discussing them or because of their recurrent nature, seemed important. We also began with a set of codes taken roughly from the interview guide since we derived the topics from our research questions about issues relevant to drug use during pregnancy.

Memoing

The interview was memoed after coding, at which time we made theoretical and methodological notes about the data.

Basically, we addressed the question "What is going on here?" The memos varied in length and often contained direct quotes from interviews that would ultimately be quoted in publications. The memoing was also done on the computer and the memos filed according to the code to which they corresponded. Memo making is the hallmark of the method used in this study. While coding the data for prominent dimensions and certainly afterward, we made theoretical memos to be used in the analysis (Glaser 1978).

Interview Guide Structuring

After approximately five interviews had been transcribed, coded, and memoed, the research team read all the memos and, based upon what they contained, scrutinized the interview guide for new areas of investigation. In this way, we probed areas that were emerging as important and put less emphasis on areas that did not elicit much response and therefore did not seem salient to the phenomena.

Weekly Analysis Sessions

Each week the entire research team convened to discuss methodological and substantive issues. In the early stages of the project, our concern was recruitment, interviewing, and instrument revision. Once we were fully under way, we began to concentrate on substantive aspects of the data we had collected. During these weekly sessions we discussed, analyzed, and conceptualized our data and then readied ourselves for the process of presenting our findings.

Presentation of Findings

Throughout the study's duration, perhaps no single issue was as divisive as how to present our findings. As we have already noted, each member of the research team came from a different scholarly background. Some differences were substantive, others historical. We shared a strong commitment to influencing policy to benefit the study participants. Only the method by which to accomplish this goal was in contention.

The Argument

The younger members of the research team, who had recently been exposed to postmodern thought through sociology or anthropology, were sensitive to the distinctions between researcher and researched (Fine 1994). Those of us in this group insisted on positioning ourselves not as experts but as co-investigators with the subjects (Fontana and Frey 1994). We cited Denzin (1994) to argue for interpretation through thick description:

> An event or process can be neither interpreted nor understood until it has been well described. However, the age of "objective" description is over. We are, as Lather (1991:91) argues, the age of inscription. Writers create their own situation, inscribed versions of the realities they describe. . . . A thin description simply reports facts, independent of intentions or circumstances. A thick description, in contrast, gives the context of an experience, states the intentions and meanings that organized the experience, and reveals the experience as a process. Out of this process arises a text's claim for truth, or its verisimilitude. (505)

Hawkesworth (1989), Clough (1992), and Fine (1992) were used to argue for maintaining the integrity of the phenomenon we studied by preserving interview texts completely.

The older (the reader should pardon the expression) members of the research team took issue with the complete preservation of text. Although we acknowledged the importance of disclosing our own autobiographies before or simultaneous to interpreting data, there seemed an inherent unfairness in allowing participants' texts to stand untouched.

In the course of writing this appendix, Rosenbaum conducted tape-recorded interviews with several members of our research team. The subject was "how we did the study," and she asked each person to tell her how she did it. While reading the transcriptions, the voices of these women, all members of our white, middle-class, well-educated team, struck her as surprisingly similar to the texts of our study participants. The women used colloquialisms; sputtered; inserted numerous "likes," "you knows," and "wells"; and started, stopped, and forgot what they were going to say midsentence. She was struck by the contrast between their spoken words and written work: the former composed their "texts," while the latter were carefully crafted, revised, and polished. If one of our goals was to ameliorate the distinctions between researcher and researched, the presentation of raw text right next to the edited versions seemed unfair. Ironically, as evidenced by Rosenbaum's interviews with the interviewers, the differences were in form (writing versus speaking) rather than content. If interviewees had had the opportunity to formally write their accounts or if we simply dictated our thoughts without editing and rethinking, the differences between us would seem less stark on paper. Nevertheless, findings/data are presented in the form of text, and analysis is painstakingly thought out and written. Therefore, it seemed to us that light editing of quotations (cleaning up extraneous words from texts to facilitate reading, just as we are doing as we edit this chapter) evens out, to the extent possible, the researchers' writing and the study participants' words.

The Compromise

Ultimately, we made the "usual compromise":

> Generally, investigators in the social sciences make those modifications in the quotation excerpts they present that they believe make the excerpts easier to grasp but that they are certain have no effect on the respondent's meaning. They are likely to permit themselves to eliminate words, sentences, and paragraphs—and also, most of the time, their own questions—in order to achieve a more compact statement. (Weiss 1994, 193)

Our findings are presented with the purpose of delivering a thick description of the experience of the pregnant woman who uses drugs. Throughout the book we offer detailed cases and almost verbatim words from study participants. All real names were changed to fictitious names for purposes of confidentiality. Our interpretations reveal our own perspectives, biases, and autobiographies. We admit, however, that for the purpose of fairness and better reading, we modified—just a little—the direct quotations. In this way, we believe we have used the PAD Project data to produce a book that best depicts the experience of these 120 women who so generously gave their time to work with us in this difficult but important undertaking.

Appendix 2

PAD Project Participants

Pseudonym	Ethnicity	Age	Stage	Drug of Choice
Abby	White	33	1	Heroin
Abigail	Latina	24	3	Heroin
Aisha	White	31	3	Heroin
Alexa	African American	23	1	Crack
Alice	Filipina	32	3	Crack
Amanda	African American	27	2	Crack
Amber	African American	35	2	Cocaine
Amy	Latina	28	1	Crack
Andrea	African American	25	1	Crack
Annie	White	23	2	Speed, crack
Antonia	White	35	3	Heroin
Ashley	African American	28	1	Heroin
Athena	African American	29	3	Crack
Aviva	White	23	1	Heroin
Beatrice	African American	27	2	Cocaine, heroin
Becky	White	26	1	Crack
Bertha	White	31	3	Heroin
Beth	White	29	3	Heroin
Bianca	African American	33	2	Heroin
Bivette	Creole	36	1	Heroin, speed
Bridget	African American	34	3	Crack
Bronwen	African American	35	3	Crack
Chandra	White	40	1	Heroin
Chelsea	African American	26	2	Crack
Cheryll	White	38	1	Heroin, cocaine, speed
Chloe	African American	24	2	Crack
Christine	African American	26	1	Cocaine, crack
Christy	African American	34	1	Crack
Clara	White	32	2	Heroin
Connie	African American	22	2	Crack
Courtney	African American	30	1	Crack
Darleen	African American	22	1	Crack
Dawn	Latina	30	3	Heroin, crack
Denise	African American	23	1	Crack

Pseudonym	Ethnicity	Age	Stage	Drug of Choice
Diane	African American	29	2	Heroin
Donna	African American	30	1	Crack
Doris	African American	24	2	Crack
Elaine	African American	20	2	Crack
Eleanor	White	24	3	Heroin
Eliza	African American	29	2	Codeine
Emily	White	32	1	Speed
Erin	White	37	1	Crack
Ethel	Latina	29	3	Crack
Evania	Latina	33	1	Heroin
Fara	White	34	3	Heroin
Franny	African American	31	2	Crack
Gia	African American	27	3	Crack
Gladys	Latina	26	1	Heroin
Glorietta	African American	40	3	Heroin, crack
Haley	White	38	3	Heroin
Heather	White	39	2	Crack, cocaine
Henrietta	White	37	3	Heroin, methadone
Hilary	African American	27	2	Crack
Holly	White	29	2	Heroin
Ingrid	White	25	3	Heroin
Jackie	African American	30	3	Crack
Jamie	African American	32	2	Crack
Jamila	White	37	3	Heroin
Jenny	African American	29	1	Crack
Jessica	African American	35	1	Crack
Jessie	African American	33	3	Crack
Jocylene	African American	26	2	Crack
Joelle	Hawaiian	22	2	Crack
Judith	African American	27	3	Heroin, crack
Julia	White	42	1	Heroin
Juliette	African American	30	3	Crack
Junelle	White	36	2	Heroin
Karene	African American	34	1	Crack
Kathy	African American	47	1	Heroin, cocaine, crack
Kelly	African American	35	1	Crack
Krista	White	29	2	Heroin, speed
Kristen	African American	22	1	Crack
Laura	African American	29	2	Heroin, crack
Lauren	White	19	2	Speed
Lavinia	White	32	3	Heroin
Lilly	Asian	35	1	Heroin
Lindley	African American	21	1	Crack
Liz	Asian	28	1	Heroin
Logan	White	31	2	Speed
Lola	African American	23	3	Crack

Pseudonym	Ethnicity	Age	Stage	Drug of Choice
Lorraine	White	38	1	Speed
Lucy	African American	30	3	Crack
Maria	African American	34	2	Crack
Mariah	African American	22	2	Crack
Marilyn	African American	30	3	Crack
Marlene	African American	20	2	Crack
Maya	White	27	3	Heroin
Melanie	Samoan	33	2	Heroin
Mindy	African American	29	3	Heroin
Moira	African American	23	2	Crack
Molly	White	23	1	Speed
Nancy	African American	27	3	Crack
Naomi	White	29	1	Heroin
Nelly	African American	34	3	Crack
Oprah	African American	32	3	Crack
Pamela	White	39	1	Speed
Patty	African American	31	3	Crack
Paula	White	30	3	Crack
Peggy	African American	34	2	Crack
Phoebe	African American	20	2	Crack
Rhoda	African American	30	1	Crack
Rita	White	27	2	Heroin
Rochelle	White	31	1	Heroin
Rosa	White	29	3	Heroin
Roseanne	White	30	1	Heroin
Sally	White	31	3	Speed
Sandra	African American	23	3	Cocaine
Sandra	African American	32	2	Crack, cocaine
Sasha	African American	24	2	Crack
Sidney	White	31	2	Heroin
Susie	African American	27	3	Crack
Sylvia	African American	36	2	Crack
Tanya	White	29	2	Heroin
Terra	African American	28	1	Cocaine, crack
Thelma	African American	25	3	Crack
Tiffany	White	24	2	Speed
Twyla	White	36	3	Heroin
Vanessa	Latina	24	2	Crack
Veronica	Latina	34	1	Heroin
Vicky	African American	31	1	Crack

Notes

1 Wayward Wombs

1. All the proper names used in this book are pseudonyms to protect confidentiality. Please refer to appendix 2 for information regarding the women's age, ethnicity, stage in pregnancy, and drug of choice.

4 Harm Perception and Harm Reduction

1. Three other women told us at the time of their interview that they planned to talk with a health professional about termination. We recruited women who used drugs while pregnant and who were currently pregnant or within six months of delivery. Therefore, in all probability our recruitment methods excluded drug-using women who opted to abort.
2. Due to our ethnographic sampling methods, the racial breakdown of this sample is in no way representative of the population of pregnant crack users or pregnant users of any other drugs.
3. See also Margaret Kearney, Katherine Irwin, Sheigla Murphy, and Marsha Rosenbaum, "Damned if You Do, Damned if You Don't: Crack Users and Prenatal Care," *Contemporary Drug Problems* 22 (Winter 1995).

5 The Final Showdown: Birth and Delivery

1. California law states that "any indication of maternal substance abuse shall lead to an assessment of the needs of the mother and child pursuant to Sec. 10901 of the Health and Safety Code. If other factors are present that indicate risk to a child, then a report shall be made. However, a report based on risk to a child which relates solely to the inability of the parent to provide the child with regular care due to the parent's substance abuse shall be made only to county welfare departments and not to law enforcement agencies" ("Effect of Positive Toxicology Screen at Time of Delivery of Infant," article 2.5 of *Child Abuse and Neglect Reporting Act*, sec.

11165.13). Furthermore, health practitioners are bound by California law to report cases of child abuse to a child protective agency: "Except as provided in subdivision (b), any child care custodian, health practitioner, or employee of a child protective agency who has knowledge of or observes a child in his or her professional capacity or within the scope of his or her employment whom he or she knows or reasonably suspects has been the victim of child abuse shall report the known or suspected instance of child abuse to a child protective agency immediately or as soon as practically possible by telephone and shall prepare and send a written report thereof within 36 hours of receiving the information concerning the incident" (sec. 11166).

6 "Not Good Enough to Be Pregnant": Conclusions and Policy Implications

1. Not all theorists agree with this social construction of mothering vis-à-vis feminine identity and adult status. But in the social worlds of our interviewees, *not* being a mother was a situation to be explained. Motherhood was such an expected part of women's lives that "childless women [were] also defined in relation to childbearing ... as failed childbearers or selfish individualists who have chosen to remain childless" (Phoenix and Woollet 1991).

Appendix I Women Talking to Women: Methodological and Theoretical Perspectives

1. Interviewees in stage 1 were required to provide appropriate documentation of pregnancy. If a woman suspected that she was pregnant and did not have documentation, we referred her for testing.
2. If the mother did not have custody of the child or if the child was unavailable or deceased, we relied on verification from friends, neighbors, or official documents (for example, birth certificates, death certificates, and CPS reports).

References

Abelson, H. I., and J. D. Miller. 1985. "A Decade of Trends in Cocaine Use in the Household Population." In *Cocaine Use in America: Epidemiological and Clinical Perspectives,* edited by N. J. Kozel and E. H. Adams. NIDA Research Monograph 61. Rockville, Md.: National Institute on Drug Abuse.

Abramovitz, M. 1988. *Regulating the Lives of Women.* Boston: South End.

Acker, D., B. P. Sachs, K. J. Tracey, and W. E. Wise. 1983. "Abruptio Placentae Associated with Cocaine Use." *American Journal of Obstetrics and Gynecology* 146, no. 2: 220–21.

Adams, E. H., and J. Durrell. 1984. "Cocaine: A Growing Public Health Problem." In *Cocaine: Pharmacology, Effects and Treatment of Abuse,* edited by J. Grabowski. NIDA Research Monograph 50 Rockville, Md.: National Institute on Drug Abuse.

Amaro, H., L. E. Fried, C. Howard, and B. Zuckerman. 1990. "Violence During Pregnancy and Substance Use." *American Journal of Public Health* 80, no. 5: 575–579.

Arif, A., and J. Westermeyer, eds. 1990. "Methadone in the Management of Opiod Dependence: Programs and Policies Around the World." In *The World Health Organization.* New York: Praeger.

Armstrong, B., A. McDonald, and M. Sloan. 1992. "Cigarette, Alcohol, and Coffee Consumption and Spontaneous Abortion." *American Journal of Public Health* 82, no. 1: 85–87.

Babbie, E. 1986. *The Practice of Social Research.* Belmont, Calif.: Wadsworth.

Baldwin, D., M. Breht, G. Monahan, K. Annon, J. Wellisch, and D. Anglin. 1995. "Perceived Need for Treatment among Pregnant and Nonpregnant Women Arrestees." *Journal of Psychoactive Drugs* 27, no. 4: 389–99.

Balisy, S. 1987. "Maternal Substance Abuse: The Need to Provide Legal Protection for the Fetus." *Southern California Law Review* 60: 1209–38.

Barth, R. 1991. "Crack Babies Grow Up." *Social Welfare* 4, no. 1: 11.

Becker, H. 1963. *Outsiders.* New York: Free Press.

———. 1970. *Sociological Work.* Chicago: Aldine.

Beckett, K. 1995. "Fetal Rights and 'Crack Moms':" Pregnant Women in the War on Drugs." *Contemporary Drug Problems* 22, no. 4: 587–607.

Beckman, L. 1978. "The Self-Esteem of Women Alcoholics." *Journal of Studies on Alcohol* 39: 491–98.

Besharov, D. 1990. "Crack Children in Foster Care." *Children Today* 35 (July–August): 21–25.

Biernacki, P., and D. Waldorf. 1981. "Snowball Sampling: Problems, Techniques and Chain-Referral Sampling." *Sociological Methods and Research* 10, no. 2: 141–63. Blakeslee, S. 1989. "Crack's Toll Among Babies: A Joyless View, Even of Toys." *New York Times*, 17 September, sec. 1, p. 1.

Blinick, G. 1971. "Fertility of Narcotics Addicts and Effects of Addiction on the Offspring." *Social Biology* 18: 34–39.

Blinick, G., C. Inturrisi, E. Jerez, et al. 1975. "Methadone Assays in Pregnant Women and Progeny." *American Journal Obstetrics and Gynecology* 1: 617–19.

Blinick, G., E. Jerez, and R. Wallach. 1973. "Methadone Maintenance, Pregnancy and Progeny." *Journal of the American Medical Association* 225: 447–79.

Blinick, G., C. Wallach, and E. Jerez. 1969. "Pregnancy in Narcotics Addicts Treated by Medical Withdrawal." *American Journal of Obstetrics and Gynecology* 105: 997–1003.

Blumer, H. 1969. *Symbolic Interactionism*. Englewood Cliffs, N.J.: Prentice Hall.

Bowman, C., and A. Rojas. 1995. "Home Is Not So Sweet." *San Francisco Chronicle*, 3 April, secs. A1 and A4.

Burks, J. 1992. "Factors in the Utilization of Prenatal Services by Low-Income Pregnant Women." *Nurse Practitioner* 17, no. 4: 34–46, 49.

Carr, J. 1975. "Drug Patterns Among Drug-Addicted Mothers: Incidence, Variance in Use and Effects on Children." *Pediatric Annals* (July): 66–77.

Charon, J. 1995. *Symbolic Interactionism: An Introduction, An Interpretation, An Integration*. Englewood Cliffs, N.J.: Prentice Hall.

Chasnoff, I. 1988. "Cocaine: Effects on Pregnancy and the Neonate." In *Drugs, Alcohol, Pregnancy and Parenting*, edited by I. J. Chasnoff. Boston: Kluwer Academic Publishers.

———. 1989. "Drug Use and Women: Establishing a Standard of Care." *Annals of New York Academy of Sciences* 562: 208–210.

———. 1992. Keynote address. Conference on Pregnancy and Drug Use, Stanford University, March.

Chasnoff, I., W. Burns, S. Schnoll, and K. Burns. 1985. "Cocaine Use in Pregnancy." *New England Journal of Medicine* 313: 666–69.

Chasnoff, I., D. Griffith, C. Freier, and J. Murray. 1992. "Cocaine/Polydrug Use During Pregnancy: Two-Year Followup." *Pediatrics* 89: 284–89.

Chasnoff, I., H. Landress, and M. Barrett. 1990. "The Prevalence of Illicit-Drug or Alcohol Use During Pregnancy and Discrepancies in Mandatory Reporting in Pinellas County, Florida." *New England Journal of Medicine* 322, no. 17: 1202–6.

Chavkin, W. 1990. "Drug Addiction and Pregnancy: Policy Crossroads." *American Journal of Public Health* 80, no. 4: 483–87.

———. 1991. "Mandatory Treatment for Drug Use During Pregnancy." *Journal of the American Medical Association* 266, no. 11: 1556–61.

Chavkin, W., M. Allen, and M. Oberman. 1991. "Drug Abuse and Pregnancy: Some Questions on Public Policy, Clinical Management, and Maternal and Fetal Rights." *Birth* 18, no. 2: 107–2.

Chavkin, W., and S. Kandall. 1990. "Between a 'Rock' and a Hard Place: Perinatal Drug Abuse." *Pediatrics* 85: 223–25.

Chodorow, N. 1978. *The Reproduction of Mothering: Psychoanalysis and the Sociology of Gender.* Berkeley: University of California Press.

Clark, D., L. Keith, R. Pildes, et al. 1974. "Drug Dependent Obstetric Patients." *Journal of Obstetrics and Gynecological Nursing* 3: 17–20.

Clayton, R., H. Voss, C. Robbins, and W. Skinner. 1985. "Gender Preferences in Drug Use: An Epidemiological Perspective." NIDA Research Monograph 65. Rockville, Md.: National Institute on Drug Abuse.

Clough, P. 1992. *The End(s) of Ethnography: From Realism to Social Criticism.* Newbury Park, Calif.: Sage.

Cohen, S., and L. Neumann. 1973. "Methadone Maintenance During Pregnancy." *American Journal of Diseases of Children* 6: 445–446.

Coles, C., K. Platzman, I. Smith, M. James, and A. Falek. 1992. "Effects of Cocaine and Alcohol Use in Pregnancy on Neonatal Growth and Neurobehavioral Status." *Neurotoxicology and Teratology* 14: 23–33.

Connaughton, J., L. Finnegan, J. Schut, and J. Emich. 1974. "Current Concepts in the Management of the Pregnant Opiate Addict." Paper presented at the National Institute on Drug Abuse Perinatal Conference, Nashville, September. Also in *International Journal of Addictive Diseases* (1975).

Connaughton, J., D. Reeser, J. Schut, and L. Finnegan. 1977. "Perinatal Addiction: Outcome and Management." *American Journal of Obstetrics and Gynecology* 9: 679–86.

Cuskey, W., L. Berger, and J. Densen-Gerber. 1977. "Issues in the Treatment of Female Addiction: A Review and Critique of the Literature." *Contemporary Drug Problems* 6, no. 3: 307–71.

Daghestani, A. 1988. "Psychsocial Characteristics of Pregnant Women Addicts in Treatment." In *Drugs, Alcohol, Pregnancy and Parenting,* edited by I. Chasnoff. Boston: Kluwer Academic Publishers.

Davis, R., and J. Chappel. 1973. "Pregnancy in the Context of Narcotic Addiction and Methadone Maintenance." Proceedings of the Fifth National Conference on Methadone Treatment, Washington, D.C., March.

Denzin, N. 1994. "The Art and Politics of Interpretation." In *Handbook of Qualitative Research*, edited by N. Denzin and Y. Lincoln. Thousand Oaks, Calif.: Sage.

Denzin, N., and Y. Lincoln. 1994. "Introduction: Entering the Field of Qualitative Research." In *Handbook of Qualitative Research*, edited by N. Denzin and Y. Lincoln. Thousand Oaks, Calif.: Sage.

Deren, S. 1986. "Children of Substance Abusers: A Review of the Literature." *Journal of Substance Abuse Treatment* 3: 77–94.

Duster, T. 1970. *The Legislation of Morality: Laws, Drugs and Moral Judgment.* New York: Free Press.

Economist. 1989. "Crack Babies," 1 April, p. 28.

Estes, C., L. Gerard, J. Zones, and J. Swan. 1984. *Political Economy, Health, and Aging.* Boston: Little, Brown.

Ethnograph. 1989. A qualitative data management program. Littleton, Colo.: Qualis Research Associates.

Fagan, J. 1995. "Women and Drugs Revisited: Female Participation in the Cocaine Economy." *Journal of Drug Issues* 24: 179–225.

Feldman, H. 1968. "Ideological Supports to Becoming and Remaining a Heroin Addict." *Journal of Health and Social Behavior* 9: 131–39.

Feldstein, P. 1988. *Health Care Economics.* New York: Wiley.

Field, P., P. Marck, G. Anderson, and K. McGeary. 1994. Introduction. In *Uncertain Motherhood: Negotiating the Risks of the Childbearing Years.* Thousand Oaks, Calif.: Sage.

Fine, M. 1992. "Passions, Politics and Power: Feminist Research Possibilities." In *Disruptive Voices*, edited by M. Fine. Ann Arbor: University of Michigan Press.

———. 1994. "Working the Hyphens: Reinventing Self and Other in Qualitative Research." In *Handbook of Qualitative Research*, edited by N. Denzin and Y. Lincoln. Thousand Oaks, Calif.: Sage.

Fink, J. 1990. "Reported Effects of Crack and Cocaine on Infants." *Youth Law News* 11, no. 1: 37–39.

Finkelstein, N. 1994. "Treatment Issues for Alcohol and Drug Dependent Pregnant and Parenting Women." *Health and Social Work* 19, no. 1: 7–15.

Finnegan, L. 1975. "Narcotics Dependence in Pregnancy." *Journal of Psychedelic Drugs* 7 (July–September): 3.

———. 1978. "Drug Dependence in Pregnancy: Clinical Management of Mother and Child." A manual for medical professionals and paraprofessionals prepared for the National Institute on Drug Abuse, Services Research Branch. Washington, D. C.: Government Printing Office.

———. 1979. "Women in Treatment." In *Handbook on Drug Abuse,* edited by R. Dupont, A. Goldstein, and J. O'Donnell. Rockville, Md.: National Institute on Drug Abuse.

———. 1988. "Drug Addiction and Pregnancy: The Newborn." In *Drugs, Alcohol, Pregnancy and Parenting*, edited by I. J. Chasnoff. Boston: Kluwer Academic Publishers.

Finnegan, L., J. Connaughton, and J. Emich. 1972. "Comprehensive Care of the Pregnant Addict and Its Effect on Maternal and Infant Outcome." *Contemporary Drug Problems* 1: 795.

———. 1973. "Abstinence Score in the Treatment of Infants of Drug Dependent Mothers." *Pediatric Research* 7: 319.

Fishburne, P., H. Abelson, and I. Cisin. 1979. "National Survey on Drug Abuse: Main Findings." EW-EW Publication 80–976. Rockville, Md.: National Institute on Drug Abuse.

Fisher, M., B. Ewigman, J. Campbell, R. Benfer, L. Furbee, L., and S. Zweig. 1991. "Cognitive Factors Influencing Women to Seek Care during Pregnancy." *Family Medicine* 23: 443–46.

Fontana, A., and J. Frey. 1994. "Interviewing: The Art of Science." In *Handbook of Qualitative Research*, edited by N. Denzin and Y. Lincoln. Thousand Oaks, Calif.: Sage.

Geertz, C. 1973. *The Interpretation of Cultures*. New York: Harpers.

Gerstein, D. R., and H. J. Harwood, eds. 1990–92. *Treatment of Drug Problems*. 2 vols. Washington, D.C.: National Academy Press.

Gillman, D. 1989. "The Children of Crack." *Washington Post*, 31 July, sec. D, p. 3.

Glass, L. 1974. "Narcotic Withdrawal in the Newborn Infant." *Journal of the National Medical Association* 66: 117–20.

Glaser, B. 1978. *Theoretical Sensitivity*. Mill Valley, Calif.: Sociology Press.

Glaser, B., and A. Strauss. 1970. *The Discovery of Grounded Theory: Strategies for Qualitative Research*. Chicago: Aldine.

Glasser, I., and L. Siegel. 1997. "When Constitutional Rights Seem Too Extravagant to Endure: The Crack Scare's Impact on Civil Rights and Liberties." In *Crack in America: Demon Drugs and Social Justice*, edited by C. Reinarman and H. Levine. Berkeley: University of California Press.

Goetz, J., and M. LeCompte. 1984. *Ethnography and Qualitative Design in Educational Research*. Orlando, Fla.: Academic Press.

Goffman, E. 1963. *Stigma: Notes on the Management of a Spoiled Identity*. Englewood Cliffs, N.J.: Prentice Hall.

Gold, R., A. Kenney, and S. Singh. 1987. "Paying for Maternity Care in the United States." *Family Planning Perspectives* 19: 190–206.

Gomby, D., and P. Shiono. 1991. "Estimating the Number of Drug Exposed Infants." *Future of Children* 1, no. 1: 17–25.

Greene, M., S. Nightingale, and R. DuPont. 1975. "Evolving Patterns of Drug Abuse." *Annals of Internal Medicine* 83: 402–11.

Gusfield, J. 1981. *The Culture of Public Problems: Drinking, Driving, and the Symbolic Order*. Chicago: University of Chicago Press.

Habel, L., K. Kaye, and J. Lee. 1990. "Trends in Reporting of Maternal Drug Abuse and Infant Mortality Among Drug-Exposed Infants in New York City." *Women and Health* 16: 41–59.

Hall, J., and P. Stevens. 1991. "Rigor in Feminist Research." *Advances in Nursing Science* 13, no. 3: 16–29.

Harper, R., G. Solish, H. Purow, E. Sand, and W. Panepinto. 1974. "The Effect of a Methadone Treatment Program Upon Pregnant Heroin Addicts and their Newborn Infants." *Pediatrics* 54: 300–305.

Harrison, M. 1991. "Drug Addiction in Pregnancy: The Interface of Science, Emotion, and Social Policy." *Journal of Substance Abuse Treatment* 8: 261–68.

Hawkesworth, M. 1989. "Knowers, Knowing, Known: Feminist Theory and Claims of Truth." *Signs* 14: 533–57.

Hinds, M. D. 1990. "The Instincts of Parenthood Become Part of Crack's Toll." *New York Times,* 17 March.

Humphries, D. 1999. *Crack Moms.* Columbus: Ohio State University Press.

Humphries, D., J. Dawson, V. Cronin, P. Keating, C. Wisniewski, and J. Eichfeld. 1992. "Mothers and Children, Drugs and Crack: Reactions to Maternal Drug Dependency." In *The Criminalization of a Woman's Body,* edited by C. Feinman. New York: Haworth.

Inciardi, J. 1986. *The War on Drugs: Heroin, Cocaine, Crime and Public Policy.* Palo Alto, Calif.: Mayfield.

Irwin, J. 1970. *The Felon.* Englewood Cliffs, N.J.: Prentice Hall.

Irwin, K. 1995. "Ideology, Pregnancy and Drugs: Differences Between Crack-Cocaine, Heroin and Methamphetamine Users." *Contemporary Drug Problems* 22, no. 4.

Jessup, M., and J. Green. 1987. "Treatment of the Pregnant Alcohol Dependent Woman." *Journal of Psychoactive Drugs* 19: 193–203.

Johnson, C. 1994. "Tenants Say Geneva Towers Makes Them Sick." *San Francisco Chronicle,* 1 July, A21.

Johnston, L., J. Bachman, and P. O'Malley. 1984. *Highlights from Student Drug Use in America, 1975–1984.* Washington, D.C.: National Institute on Drug Abuse, U.S. Department of Health and Human Services.

Kaestner, E., B. Frank, R. Marel, and J. Schmeidler. 1986. "Substance Abuse Among Females: Catching Up with the Males." *Advances in Alcohol and Substance Abuse* 5, no. 3: 29–49.

Kalton, G. 1983. *Introduction to Survey Sampling.* Beverly Hills, Calif.: Sage.

Kandall, S., S. Albin, J. Lowinson, B. Berle, A. Eidelman, and L. Gartner. 1976. "Differential Effects of Maternal Heroin and Methadone Use on Birthweight." *Pediatrics* 58: 681–85.

Kearney, M., K. Irwin, S. Murphy, and M. Rosenbaum. 1995. "Crack Users and Prenatal Care." *Contemporary Drug Problems* 22, no. 4: 639–62.

Kearney, M., S. Murphy, and M. Rosenbaum. 1994a. "Learning by Losing: Sex and Fertility on Crack Cocaine." *Qualitative Health Research* 4, no. 2: 142–62.

———. 1994b. "Mothering on Crack Cocaine: A Grounded Theory Analysis." *Social Science and Medicine* 38, no. 20: 351–61.

Koren, G., H. Shear, K. Graham, and T. Einarson. 1989. "Bias Against the Null Hypothesis: The Reproductive Hazards of Cocaine." *Lancet*, 16 December, pp. 1440–42.

Krieger, S. 1991. *Social Science and the Self: Personal Essays on an Art Form.* New Brunswick, N.J.: Rutgers University Press.

Land, D., and R. Kushner. 1990. "Drug Abuse during Pregnancy in an Inner-City Hospital: Prevalence and Patterns. *Journal of the American Osteopathic Association* 90: 421–26.

Levy, S., and K. Doyle. 1974. "Attitudes Towards Women in a Drug Treatment Program." *Journal of Drug Issues* 4: 428–34.

Lieb, J., and C. Sterk-Elifson. 1995. "Crack in the Cradle: Social Policy and Reproductive Rights Among Crack Using Females." *Contemporary Drug Problems* 22, no. 4: 687–705.

Lindesmith, A. 1968. *Opiate Addiction.* Bloomington, Ind.: Principa.

Lofland, J. 1971. *Analyzing Social Settings: A Guide to Qualitative Observation and Analysis.* Belmont, Calif.: Wadsworth.

Lodge, A., M. Marcus, and C. Ramer. 1975. "Behavioral and Electro-Physiological Characteristics of the Addicted Neonate." *Addictive Disease: An International Journal* 2: 235–55.

Lutiger, B., K. Graham, T. Einarson, and G. Koren. 1991. "Relationship Between Gestational Cocaine Use and Pregnancy Outcome: A Meta-Analysis." *Teratology* 44: 405–14.

McBride, D., and R. Clayton. 1985. "Methodological Issues in the Etiology of Drug Abuse." *Journal of Drug Issues* 15, no. 4: 509–529.

McCalla, S., H. Minkoff, J. Feldman, L. Glass, and G. Valencia. 1992. "Predictors of Cocaine Use in Pregnancy." *Obstetrics and Gynecology* 79, no. 5: 641–44.

McDonald, A., B. Armstrong, and M. Sloan. 1992. "Cigarette, Alcohol, and Coffee Consumption and Prematurity." *American Journal of Public Health* 82, no. 1: 87–90.

McNulty, H. 1987. "Pregnancy Police: The Health Policy and Legal Implications of Punishing Women for Harm to their Fetuses." *New York University Review of Law and Social Change* 16: 277.

Maher, L., 1992. "Punishment and Welfare: Crack Cocaine and the Regulation of Mothering." In *The Criminalization of a Woman's Body,* edited by C. Feinman. New York: Haworth.

Martin, E. 1987. *The Woman in the Body.* Boston: Beacon.

Matza, D. 1969. *Becoming Deviant.* Englewood Cliffs, N.J.: Prentice Hall.

Mead, G. 1939. *Mind, Self and Society.* Chicago: Aldine.

Messer, K., K. Anderson, and S. Martin. 1996. "Characteristics Associated with Pregnant Women's Utilization of Substance Abuse Services." *American Journal of Drug and Alcohol Abuse* 22, no. 3: 403–422.

Michaels, B., M. Noonan, S. Hoffman, and R. Brennan. 1988. "A Treatment Model of Nursing Care for Pregnant Chemical Abusers." In *Drugs, Alcohol, Pregnancy and Parenting,* edited by I. Chasnoff. Boston: Kluwer Academic Publishers.

Miller, B., W. Downs, and M. Testa. 1989. "Spousal Violence Among Alcoholic Women as Compared to a Random Household Sample of Women." *Journal of Studies on Alcohol* 50, no. 6: 533–540.

Mondanaro, J. 1977. "Women: Pregnancy, Children and Addiction." *Journal of Psychedelic Drugs* 9, no. 1: 59–68.

———. 1988. *Treating Drug Dependent Women.* Springfield, Ill.: Lexington.

Mondanaro J., M. Wedenoja, J. Densen-Gerber, J. Elahi, M. Mason, and A. Redmond. 1982. "Sexuality and Fear of Intimacy as Barriers to Recovery for Drug Dependent Women." In *Treatment Services for Drug-Dependent Women,* vol. 2. NIDA (ADM) 82–1219. Rockville, Md.: National Institute on Drug Abuse.

Morgan, J., and L. Zimmer. 1997. "The Social Pharmacology of Smokeable Cocaine: Not All It's Cracked Up to Be." In *Crack in American: Demon Drugs and Social Justice,* edited by C. Reinarman and H. Levine. Berkeley: University of California Press.

Muraskin, R. 1991. "Mothers and Fetuses: Enter the Fetal Police." In *New Frontiers in Drug Policy,* edited by A. Trebach and K. Zeese. Washington, D.C.: Drug Policy Foundation.

Murphy, S. 1987. "Intravenous Drug Use and AIDS: Notes on the Social Economy of Needle Sharing." *Contemporary Drug Problems* 14, no. 3: 373–93.

———. Forthcoming. *They Took Myself: Women and Crack.* Philadelphia: Temple University Press.

Murphy, S., and M. Rosenbaum. 1987. "Women and Substance Abuse." Introduction to a special edition of *Journal of Psychoactive Drugs* 20, no. 4: 125–28.

Nadelmann, E., P. Cohen, U. Locher, G. Stimson, A. Wodak, and E. Drucker. 1994. "The Harm Reduction Approach to Drug Control: International Progress." Working paper. New York: Lindesmith Center.

Naeye, R., W. Blanc, W. Leblanc, and M. Khatamee. 1973. "Fetal Complications of Maternal Heroin Addiction: Abnormal Growth, Infection and Episodes of Stress." *Journal of Pediatrics* 83: 1055–61.

Naeye, R., B. Ladis, and J. Drage. 1976. "Sudden Infant Death Syndrome." *American Journal of Diseases of Children* 130: 7–10.

National Institute on Drug Abuse (NIDA). 1987. "Highlights: 1985 National Household Survey on Drug Abuse." Washington, D.C.: Government Printing Office.

Navarro, V. 1986. *Crisis, Health, and Medicine: A Social Critique.* New York: Tavistock.

Newald, I. 1986. "Cocaine Infants." *Hospitals* 60: 76.

Newman, R. G. 1974. "Pregnancies of Methadone Patients." *New York State Journal of Medicine* 1: 52–54.

Norton-Hawk, M. 1994. "How Social Policies Make Matters Worse: The Case of Maternal Substance Abuse." *Journal of Drug Issues* 24, no. 3: 517–26.

Notman, M., and C. Nadelson. 1982. "Changing Views of the Relationship between Femininity and Reproduction." In *The Woman Patient: Concepts of Femininity and the Life Cycle,* edited by C. Nadelson and M. Notman. New York: Plenum.

Oakley, A. 1980. *Women Confined: Towards a Sociology of Childbirth.* Oxford: Robertson.

———. 1981. "Interviewing Women: A Contradiction in Terms." In *Doing Feminist Research,* edited by H. Roberts. London: Routledge and Kegan Paul.

O'Connor, J. 1973. *The Fiscal Crisis of the State.* New York: St. Martin's.

Olesen, V. 1994. "Feminisms and Models of Qualitative Research." In *Handbook of Qualitative Research,* edited by N. Denzin and Y. Lincoln. Thousand Oaks, Calif.: Sage.

Ostrea, E., C. Chavez, and M. Strauss. 1976. "A Study of Factors That Influence the Severity of Neonatal Narcotic Withdrawal." *Journal of Pediatrics* 88: 642–45.

Paltrow, L. 1992. "Criminal Prosecutions Against Pregnant Women." National update and overview. Reproductive Freedom Project, American Civil Liberties Union Foundation, April.

Pascall, G. 1986. *Social Policy: A Feminist Analysis.* London: Tavistock.

Patterson, E., M. Freese, and R. Goldenberg. 1990. "Seeking Safe Passage: Utilizing Health Care during Pregnancy." *Image* 22: 27–31.

Pettiti, D., and C. Coleman. 1990. "Cocaine and the Risk of Low Birth Weight. *American Journal of Public Health* 80: 25–28.

Phoenix, A., and A. Woollet. 1991. "Motherhood: Social Constructions, Politics and Psychology." In *Motherhood: Meanings, Practices and Ideologies,* edited by A. Phoenix, A. Woollet, and Eva Lloyd. London: Sage.

Poland, M., M. Dombrowski, J. Ager, and R. Sokol. 1993. "Punishing Pregnant Drug Users: Enhancing the Flight from Care." *Drug and Alcohol Dependence* 31: 199–203.

Pope, D., N. Quinn, and N. Wyer. 1990. "The Ideology of Mothering: Disruption and Reproduction of Patriarchy." *Signs* 15, no. 3: 441–46.

Preble, E., and J. Casey. 1969. "Taking Care of Business: The Heroin User's Life on the Street." *International Journal of the Addictions* 4: 1–24.

Quadagno, J. 1987. "Theories of the Welfare State." *Annual Review of Sociology* 13: 109–28.

Racine, A., T. Joyce, and R. Anderson. 1993. "The Association between Prenatal Care and Birth Weight among Women Exposed to Cocaine in New York City." *Journal of the American Medical Association* 270: 1581–86.

Rajegowda, B., L. Glass, H. Evans, G. Maso, D. Swartz, and W. LeBlanc. 1972. "Methadone Withdrawal in Newborn Infants." *Journal of Pediatrics* 81, no. 3: 532–34.

Ramer, C., and A. Lodge. 1975. "Clinical and Developmental Characteristics of Infants of Mothers on Methadone Maintenance." *Addictive Diseases* 2: 227–33.

Raskin, V. 1992. "Maternal Bereavement in the Perinatal Substance Abuser." *Journal of Substance Abuse Treatment* 9: 149–52.

Reddy, A., R. Harper, and G. Stern. 1971. "Observation of Heroin and Methadone Withdrawal in the Newborn." *Journal of Pediatrics* 48: 353–58.

Reed, B. 1987. "Developing Women-Sensitive Drug Dependence Treatment Services: Why So Difficult?" *International Journal of the Addictions* 20, no. 1: 13–62.

Reed, B. 1991. "Linkages: Battering, Sexual Assault, Incest, Child Sexual Abuse, Teen Pregnancy, Dropping Out of School and the Alcohol and Drug Connection." *Alcohol and Drugs Are Women's Issues* 1: 130–50.

Reed, B., J. Kovach, N. Bellows, and R. Moise. 1980. "The Many Faces of Addicted Women: Implications for Treatment and Future Research." In *Drug Dependence and Alcohol*, edited by A. Schechter. New York: Plenum.

Regan, D., L. O'Malley, and L. Finnegan. 1982. "The Incidence of Violence in the Lives of Pregnant Drug-Dependent Women." *Pediatric Research* 16, no. 77: 330.

Reinarman, C., and H. Levine. 1989. "The Crack Attack: Politics and Media in America's Latest Drug Scare." In *Images and Issues: Typifying Contemporary Social Problems*, edited by J. Best. New York: Aldine de Gruyer.

———. 1997. "Crack on Context: America's Latest Demon Drug." In *Crack in America: Demon Drugs and Social Justice*, edited by C. Reinarman and H. Levine. Berkeley: University of California Press.

Reinarman, C., D. Waldorf, S. Murphy, and H. Levine. 1997. "The Contingent Call of the Pipe." In *Crack in America: Demon Drugs and Social Justice*, edited by C. Reinarman and H. Levine. Berkeley: University of California Press.

Reinharz, S. 1992. *Feminist Methods in Social Research.* New York: Oxford University Press.

Rementeria, J., and N. Nunag. 1973. "Narcotic Withdrawal in Pregnancy." *American Journal of Obstetrics and Gynecology* 116: 1052–56.

Richardson, L. 1994. "Writing: A Method of Inquiry." In *Handbook of Qualitative Research*, edited by N. Denzin and Y. Lincoln. Thousand Oaks, Calif.: Sage.

Roberts, D. 1997. *Killing the Black Body: Race, Reproduction, and the Meaning of Liberty.* New York: Pantheon.

Robins, L., and N. Mills. 1993. "Effects of In Utero Exposure to Street Drugs." *American Journal of Public Health* 83, supplement: 9–13.

Rosenbaum, M. 1979. "Difficulties in Taking Care of Business: Women Addicts As Mothers." *American Journal of Drug and Alcohol Abuse* 6: 431–46.

———. 1981. *Women on Heroin.* New Brunswick, N.J.: Rutgers University Press.

———. 1982. "Getting on Methadone." *Contemporary Drug Problems* (Spring): 113–43.

Rosenbaum, M., and S. Murphy. 1981. "Getting the Treatment: Recycling Women Addicts." *Journal of Psychoactive Drugs* 13, no. 1: 1–13.

———. 1987. "Not the Picture of Health: Women on Methadone." *Journal of Psychoactive Drugs* 19, no. 2: 217–25.

Rosenbaum, M., S. Murphy, J. Irwin, and L. Watson. 1990. "Women and Crack: What's the Real Story?" In *Drug Prohibition and the Conscience of Nations,* edited by A. Trebach and K. Zeese. Washington, D.C.: Drug Policy Foundation.

Sable, M., J. Stockbauer, W. Schramm, and G. Land. 1990. "Differentiating the Barriers to Adequate Prenatal Care in Missouri, 1987–88." *Public Health Reports* 105: 549–55.

Salmon, P. 1985. *Living in Time: A New Look at Personal Development.* London: Dent.

Schutz, A. 1967. "Common Sense and Scientific Interpretations of Human Action." In *Collected Papers I: The Problem of Social Reality.* The Hague: Nijoff.

Shapiro, D., G. Perry, and C. Brewin. 1979. "Stress, Coping and Psychotherapy: The Foundations of a Clinical Approach." In *Psychophysiological Response to Occupational Stress,* edited by R. Cox and M. Mackay. New York: International Publishing.

Siegel, L. 1997. "The Pregnancy Police Fight the War on Drugs." In *Crack in America: Demon Drugs and Social Justice,* edited by C. Reinarman and H. Levine. Berkeley: University of California Press.

———. 1990. "The Criminalization of Pregnant and Child-Rearing Drug Users." *Drug Law Report* 2, no. 15: 169–79.

Siegel, R. 1982. "Cocaine and Sexual Dysfunction: The Curse of Mama Coca." *Journal of Psychoactive Drugs* 14, nos. 1 and 2: 71–74.

Skolnick, A. 1990. "Drug Screening in Prenatal Care Demands Objective Medical Criteria, Support Services." *Journal of the American Medical Association* 264: 309–10.

Smith, D. 1987. *The Everyday World as Problematic: A Feminist Sociology.* Boston: Northeastern University Press.

Soler, E., I. Ponsor, and J. Abod. 1976. "Women in Treatment: Client Self-Report." In *Women in Treatment: Issues and Approaches,* edited by A. Bauman et al. Arlington, Vir.: National Drug Abuse Center for Training and Resource Development.

Spradley, J. 1979. *The Ethnographic Interview.* New York: Holt, Rinehart, and Wilson.

Statzer, D., and J. Wardell. 1966. "Heroin Addiction During Pregnancy." *American Journal of Obstetrics and Gynecology* 94: 253–57.

Sterk, C. 1998. *Fast Lives: Women Who Use Crack Cocaine.* Philadelphia: Temple University Press.

Stone, M., L. Salerna, and M. Green. 1971. "Narcotic Addiction in Pregnancy." *American Journal of Obstetrics and Gynecology* 109: 716.

Strauss, A. 1987. *Qualitative Analysis for the Social Sciences.* Cambridge: University of Cambridge Press.

Strauss, A., and Corbin, J. 1990. *Basics of Qualitative Research: Grounded Theory Processes and Techniques.* Newbury Park, Calif.: Sage.

———. 1994. "Grounded Theory Methodology: An Overview." In *Handbook of Qualitative Research,* edited by N. Denzin and Y. Lincoln. Thousand Oaks, Calif.: Sage.

Sullivan, R., A. Fischbach, and F. Hornick. 1972. "Treatment of a Pregnant Opiate Addict with Oral Methadone." *Arizona Medicine* 29: 30.

Trebach, A., and K. Zeese, eds. 1990. *Drug Prohibition and the Conscience of Nations.* Washington, D.C.: Drug Policy Foundation.

Van Maanen, J. 1988. *Tales of the Field: On Writing Ethnography.* Chicago: University of Chicago Press.

Vega, W., B. Kolody, J. Hwang, and A. Noble. 1993. "Prevalence and Magnitude of Perinatal Substance Exposures in California." Reprint. *New England Journal of Medicine* 329: 850–54.

Vega, W., B. Kolody, A. Noble, J. Hwang, P. Porter, A. Bole, and J. Dimas. 1993. *Profile of Alcohol and Drug Use During Pregnancy in California, 1992.* Final report. Contract 91–00252. Sacramento: State of California, Health and Welfare Agency, Department of Alcohol and Drug Programs.

Waitzken, H. 1989. "Social Structures of Medical Oppression: A Marxist View." In *Perspectives in Medical Sociology,* edited by E. Brown. Belmont, Calif.: Wadsworth.

Waldeman, H. 1973. "Psychiatric Emergencies During Pregnancy and in the Puerperium." *Muencheuer Medizinische Wochenschrift* 115: 1039–43.

Waldorf, D. 1973. *Careers in Dope.* Englewood Cliffs, N.J.: Prentice Hall.

Waldorf, D., and P. Biernacki. 1981. "Natural Recovery from Opiate Addiction: Some Social-Psychological Processes of Untreated Recovery." *Journal of Drug Issues* 11: 61–74.

Waldorf, D., C. Reinarman, and S. Murphy. 1991. *Cocaine Changes: The Experience of Using and Quitting.* Philadelphia: Temple University Press.

Wallach, R., E. Jerez, and G. Blinick. 1969. "Pregnancy and Menstrual

Function in Narcotics Addicts Treated with Methadone, The Methadone Maintenance Treatment Program." *American Journal of Obstetrics and Gynecology* 105, no. 8: 1226–29.

Warren, C. 1988. *Gender Issues in Field Research.* Newbury Park, Calif.: Sage.

Watters, J., and P. Biernacki. 1989. "Targeted Sampling: Options for the Study of Hidden Populations." *Social Problems* 36, no. 4: 416–430.

Weimann, C., A. Berenson, and B. Landwehr. 1995. "Racial and Ethnic Correlates of Tobacco, Alcohol and Illicit Drug Use in a Pregnant Population." *Journal of Reproductive Medicine* 40, no. 8: 1566–72.

Weimann, C., A. Berenson, and V. San Miguel. 1994. "Tobacco, Alcohol and Illicit Drug Use Among Pregnant Women: Age and Racial/Ethnic Differences." *Journal of Reproductive Medicine* 39, no. 10: 1461–70.

Weiss, R. 1994. *Learning from Strangers: The Art and Method of Qualitative Interview Studies.* New York: Free Press.

Welldon, E. 1988. *Mother, Madonna, Whore: The Idealization and Denigration of Motherhood.* New York: Guilford.

Wilson, G., K. McCreary, J. Kean, and J. Baxter. 1979. "The Development of Preschool Children of Heroin-Addicted Mothers: A Controlled Study." *Pediatrics* 63: 135–41.

Worth, D. 1989. "Sexual Decision-Making and AIDS: Why Condom Promotion among Vulnerable Women Is Likely to Fail." *Studies in Family Planning* 20, no. 6: 297–307.

York, R., P. Williams, and B. Munro. 1993. "Maternal Factors That Influence Inadequate Prenatal Care." *Public Health Nursing* 10: 241–44.

Zapata, C., A. Rebolledo, E. Atalah, B. Newman, and M. King. 1992. "The Influence of Social and Political Violence on the Risk of Pregnancy Complications." *American Journal of Public Health* 82, no. 5: 685–90.

Zelson, C. 1973. "Infant of the Addicted Mother." *New England Journal of Medicine* 288: 26.

Zelson, C., S. Lee, and M. Casalino. 1973. "Neonatal Narcotic Addiction: Comparative Effects of Maternal Intake of Heroin and Methadone." *New England Journal of Medicine* 289, no. 23: 16–20.

Zelson, C., E. Rubio, and E. Wasserman. 1989. "Neonatal Narcotic Addiction: 10–Year Observation." *Pediatric Research* 25: 316–34.

Zelson, C., and J. Sook. 1973. "Neonatal Narcotic Addiction: Exposure to Heroin and Methadone." *Pediatric Research* 7, no. 4: 289–301.

Zuckerman, B. 1991. "Drug Exposed Infants: Understanding the Medical Risk." *Future of Children* 1, no. 1: 26–35.

Zuckerman, B., D. Frank, R. Hingson, H. Amaro, S. Levenson, H. Kayne, S. Parker, R. Vinci, K. Aboagye, L. Fried, H. Cabral, R. Timperi,

and H. Bauchner. 1989. "Effect of Maternal Marijuana and Cocaine Use on Fetal Growth." *New England Journal of Medicine*
320: 762–68.

Zuspan, F., J. Gumpel, A. Mejia-Zelaya, et al. 1975. "Fetal Stress from
Methadone Withdrawal." *American Journal of Obstetrics and
Gynecology* 2: 43–48.

Zweben, J., and J. Sorensen. 1988. "Misunderstandings about Methadone." *Journal of Psychoactive Drugs* 20, no. 3: 275–81.

Index

About the Authors

Sheigla Murphy, Ph.D., is a medical sociologist who has been conducting ethnographic drug research, primarily for the National Institute on Drug Abuse, for more than twenty years. Dr. Murphy is the co-author (with Dan Waldorf and Craig Reinarman) of *Cocaine Changes: The Experience of Using and Quitting* (Temple University Press, 1991) and a contributing author to *Crack in America: Demon Drugs and Social Justice* (edited by Craig Reinarman and Harry Gene Levine, University of California Press, 1997).

Marsha Rosenbaum, Ph.D., is a medical sociologist and the director of the Lindesmith Center West, a drug-policy institute in San Francisco. She has received grants for her work from the National Institute on Drug Abuse. Dr. Rosenbaum is the author of *Women on Heroin* and the co-author (with Jerome Beck) of *Pursuit of Ecstasy: The MDMA Experience.* She has written numerous scholarly articles on drug use and drug policy.